DEYR

Please return / renew by date shown.
You can renew at: **norlink.norfolk.gov.uk**
or by telephone: **0344 800 8006**
Please have your library card & PIN ready.

NORFOLK LIBRARY
AND INFORMATION SERVICE
NORFOLK ITEM

30129 076 948 711

Dementia For Dummies®

Published by: **John Wiley & Sons, Ltd.,** The Atrium, Southern Gate, Chichester, www.wiley.com

This edition first published 2015

© 2015 John Wiley & Sons, Ltd, Chichester, West Sussex.

Registered office

John Wiley & Sons Ltd, The Atrium, Southern Gate, Chichester, West Sussex, PO19 8SQ, United Kingdom

For details of our global editorial offices, for customer services and for information about how to apply for permission to reuse the copyright material in this book please see our website at www.wiley.com.

Wiley publishes in a variety of print and electronic formats and by print-on-demand. Some material included with standard print versions of this book may not be included in e-books or in print-on-demand. If this book refers to media such as a CD or DVD that is not included in the version you purchased, you may download this material at http://booksupport.wiley.com. For more information about Wiley products, visit www.wiley.com.

Designations used by companies to distinguish their products are often claimed as trademarks. All brand names and product names used in this book are trade names, service marks, trademarks or registered trademarks of their respective owners. The publisher is not associated with any product or vendor mentioned in this book.

For general information on our other products and services, please contact our Customer Care Department within the U.S. at 877-762-2974, outside the U.S. at (001) 317-572-3993, or fax 317-572-4002. For technical support, please visit www.wiley.com/techsupport.

For technical support, please visit www.wiley.com/techsupport.

A catalogue record for this book is available from the British Library.

ISBN 978-1-118-92469-3 (hardback/paperback) ISBN 978-1-118-92471-6 (ebk)

ISBN 978-1-118-92470-9 (ebk)

Printed in Great Britain by TJ International, Padstow, Cornwall

10 9 8 7 6 5 4 3 2 1

Contents at a Glance

Table of Contents

Part IV: Sorting Out Domiciliary and Longer-Term Care 233

Chapter 16: Choosing Ongoing Care for Your Loved One......... 235

Introduction

•••

*P*ick up a newspaper or turn on the television or radio, and it won't be long before you come across a reference to dementia. Either there's been a breakthrough in research, or someone famous has been diagnosed with it, or an expert has decided that some food or other, which we've previously enjoyed without a second thought, is now believed to double our risk of developing the condition.

But its media popularity isn't really that much of a shock, because dementia is on the rise. In fact, it's reckoned that every four seconds someone somewhere in the world is diagnosed with dementia, so the number of cases is rising pretty fast.

At the moment, the World Health Organization estimates that 35.6 million people have dementia across the globe, with 7.7 million cases being added every 12 months. And closer to home, the number of people in the UK with dementia is thought to be 820,000, which, according to Alzheimer's Research UK, means that 23 million of us will know a close friend or family member who has been diagnosed with it.

Sadly, those figures mean that a lot of people are, or will be, directly affected by dementia.

About This Book

The scope of this book is extremely wide ranging, covering the basics of how each of the four diseases that cause dementia develop, along with an explanation of the changes that happen in the brain to cause the disease's disabling symptoms. I look at the treatments available, both from mainstream medicine and complementary therapies, and review what works and what doesn't. Then sections give tips to carers about how to handle difficult symptoms as the condition progresses, advice on when and how to make a will, and details of how to choose the right care home. Plus much more.

This book isn't necessarily designed to be read from the front cover to the final page in order – although if you want to do that, it will take you on a logical journey from finding the diagnosis to dealing sensitively with end-of-life care. Instead, each chapter is designed to stand alone. You can read the chapters just as easily in a completely random order, according to your area of interest, as in numerical order by chapter.

The main information about each topic is contained in the main text of each chapter, but you will also notice shaded boxes of text in each chapter, called sidebars. These boxes offer interesting asides, designed to complement the rest of the chapter, rather than essential information. So if a sidebar doesn't interest you, just skip it; you'll still be able to understand everything else without it.

Within this book, you may note that some web addresses break across two lines of text. If you're reading this book in print and want to visit one of these web pages, simply key in the address exactly as it's noted in the text, pretending that the line break doesn't exist. If you're reading this as an e-book, you've got it easy: just click the web address to be taken directly to the page.

Foolish Assumptions

I've written this book with everyone who has dementia or who may one day be affected by dementia in mind. It's for those who are just generally worried about dementia and want to find out more about the condition and how it develops, as well as for those currently experiencing symptoms that they think may mean they already have dementia and who want to know what they should do next. It's also for people who've already been given the diagnosis and who need advice about how to get the best care available, and for those looking after people with dementia who want to know how to be the best carers they can be.

But despite the wealth of information, I've designed this book so that you don't need to

- Have a degree in medicine or biology to understand the science stuff
- Be trained in social work to follow details of how to navigate the care and benefits system
- Be a lawyer to write the most appropriate, all-encompassing, watertight will

Everything in this book should make sense to everyone with an interest in dementia and how best to care for the people who develop it.

Icons Used in This Book

As you go through the book, you'll notice that a variety of different icons pop up in the margins. These are designed to identify information that you need to know; information that may be interesting, but which you can live without; and hints about how to understand what you're reading.

These are handy bits of information that are worth remembering because they will help you deal with problems and perhaps see them off before they arise.

These are key facts that anyone wanting to get a handle on dementia and what it's all about will want to know.

This icon flags potential dangers and pitfalls that can lead to problems when managing dementia.

This icon points out information that's interesting or in-depth but that isn't necessary for you to read.

Beyond the Book

In addition to the material in the print or e-book you're reading right now, this product also comes with some access-anywhere goodies on the web. These resources are crammed with useful summaries about everything you need to know about dementia. Check out the free cheat sheet at `http://www.dummies.com/cheatsheet/dementia` for more information about the condition and helpful reminders about the essentials of being a carer.

And you'll also find online articles at `www.dummies.com/extras/dementia`. There's one looking at the tests that doctors carry out to diagnose dementia, another on the steps you need to follow to set up a lasting power of attorney and finally an article highlighting the top tips for finding a suitable care home.

Where to Go from Here

By all means carry on reading from here in chapter order; if you do, you obviously won't go far wrong. But if you have particular needs and interests when it comes to dementia and its care then you may well want to flit about through the book.

If you want to understand the causes of dementia and the way the disease affects the brain then head to Chapter 4. If you need to grasp the difference between Alzheimer's disease, vascular dementia, Lewy body disease and fronto-temporal dementia then I discuss these in Chapter 3.

If the medical bits don't really captivate you, but you want tips about being a great carer, then you can start reading from Chapter 10. Or if you're worried you may have dementia and need to know how to have it diagnosed then you should start reading at Chapter 6.

Basically, thanks to the layout of all *For Dummies* books, the choice of how you read through this book is completely yours. But, however you decide to set off, I hope you enjoy learning more about this increasingly important subject.

Part I
Could It Be Dementia?

In this part . . .

✔ Find out what dementia actually is and the symptoms that someone may develop that lead a doctor to consider the diagnosis.

✔ Look at the main diseases that cause dementia, and at some other medical conditions whose symptoms, while similar, can be reversible with appropriate treatment.

✔ Discover the causes of the condition and the risk factors for developing it, and ways to possibly protect yourself from getting it.

✔ Explore the various stages of the disease and the symptoms to look out for as time goes on.

Chapter 1

Checking Out the Facts on Dementia

*I*f you're reading a book about dementia, you first need to understand what the term means. In my work as a family doctor I meet people with a whole heap of different ideas about what sort of condition the word 'dementia' suggests. For some, it's the diagnostic label you give to people who keep having 'senior moments' and regularly forget what they've been up to, where they put their spectacles and the names of their grandchildren. To others, it refers to people who are old and confused, have urine-drenched armchairs, and spend all day shouting at the telly and letting their friends and neighbours know exactly what they think of them.

While some of the above symptoms clearly can be part of the picture, neither of the people described fits the diagnosis. The first is probably just forgetful but otherwise well, and the second may simply be leaky and bad-tempered, with a poor sense of smell. Dementia has a very clear definition, because the diagnosis is never made lightly.

This chapter looks in detail at what dementia is and what it certainly is not.

Understanding What Dementia Is

Dementia isn't a single entity, but the result of a number of different medical conditions that affect normal brain functioning.

The World Health Organization (WHO) defines dementia thus:

> [A] syndrome – usually of a chronic or progressive nature – in which there is deterioration in cognitive function (i.e. the ability to process thought) beyond what might be expected from normal ageing. It affects memory, thinking, orientation, comprehension, calculation, learning capacity, language, and judgement. Consciousness is not affected. The impairment in cognitive function is commonly accompanied, and occasionally preceded, by deterioration in emotional control, social behaviour, or motivation.

This definition, however, still contains a fair amount of medical jargon. So I'll try to come up with a simpler, but still accurate, version by considering each of the key terms used by the WHO:

- ✔ **Syndrome:** This word describes the symptoms that are characteristic of a particular medical condition. People with the condition have most of these features but don't have to show all of them to receive the diagnosis. Thus in dementia, one person may have poor memory for shopping lists but still be able to add up the prices on the bill, while another may have problems with both memory and calculations.

- ✔ **Chronic and progressive:** These terms mean that the condition is long term and gets steadily worse with time. Many people think that the word 'chronic' means that something is severe. But while dementia may be severe for some people, it's mild in others; chronic here means long-lasting.

- ✔ **Consciousness:** Used in relation to dementia, this word takes on both of its meanings. People with dementia are both awake (as opposed to unconscious) and mentally aware of their surroundings, although what's going on around them may not always make sense and may be confusing.

So dementia can be caused by a number of diseases of the brain that lead to a collection of progressively worsening symptoms affecting a person's thought processes, mood and behaviour; eventually, the person may lose the ability to carry out the basic tasks of daily living.

Grasping What Dementia Is Not

Many myths and misunderstandings circulate about dementia. And to get a grasp of what dementia actually is, it's important to have a clear idea about what it certainly isn't. So here's a selection of some of the most common misconceptions, to help sort fact from fiction.

- ✔ **All old people get dementia.** Although the chances of developing dementia do increase as we get older, it's not a normal part of the ageing process. In fact only 1 in 14 people over the age of 65 and 1 in 6 over 80 suffer from it.

- **Dementia is the same as Alzheimer's disease.** Alzheimer's disease is just one of a number of brain diseases that lead to dementia.

- **Memory loss equals dementia.** Dementia does affect memory, but for someone to be diagnosed with the condition he needs to show many other more complex symptoms rather than simply poor memory alone.

- **Everyone with dementia becomes aggressive.** While some people with dementia can become agitated, aggression isn't a universal feature of dementia and is usually triggered by the way someone is treated or communicated with rather than being a symptom of the dementia alone.

- **A diagnosis of dementia means a person's life is over.** Despite the fact that the condition is chronic and progressive, many medical, social and psychological treatments and strategies are available to help make life as fulfilling as possible for someone with dementia, for many years.

- **Everyone with dementia ends up in a nursing home.** While one third of people with dementia do eventually need this level of intense care in the latter stages of their condition, many people are able to access enough help and support to spend the rest of their lives in their own homes.

- **My nan has dementia, so I'm going to get it too.** Some forms of dementia do have a genetic component and so may run in families, but these are in the minority. For most people, it doesn't follow that because a relative has dementia, they'll get it too. And contrary to what one patient of mine thought, you can't catch it off your nan either!

Looking at the Statistics

Now that I've excluded all the people who don't really have dementia from the discussion, I can look more accurately at what the statistics reveal about who actually has the diagnosis. And, unfortunately, the results still make rather sobering reading.

The statistics tell us that every four seconds, someone in the world is diagnosed with dementia. That's 15 people per minute, 900 per hour and 1,350 during a 90-minute game of football or an average-length Hollywood blockbuster. In fact, by the time you go to bed tonight, around another 21,600 people will have been told they have dementia in the previous 24 hours. Over the course of 12 months, that's a whopping 7.7 million new cases.

And, worse still, those people are just the tip of the diagnostic iceberg, because it's reckoned that up to six out of ten people with dementia may still be undiagnosed in the UK alone. Start adding those figures into the calculations, and the statistics start to look even more frightening.

Without being sensationalist, knowing what we're all up against is important, not only so that governments and health professionals can plan for the types of care that may be needed as the disease becomes more common, but also to enable individuals and their families to be reassured that they're by no means alone in their struggles.

According to statistics from the organisation Alzheimer's Disease International:

- Currently, 44.4 million people around the world are living with dementia.
- The number of people living with dementia is expected to double by 2030 and treble by 2050.
- Sixty-two per cent of people with dementia live in developing countries, a proportion that's expected to rise to 71 per cent by 2050.
- In economic terms, the cost of dementia care is $600 billion worldwide, which means that
    - If dementia was a country, it would be the world's 18th-largest economy, sandwiched between Turkey and Indonesia.
    - If dementia was a multinational company, it would be the biggest in the world, out-grossing both Walmart and Exxon Mobile.
- The increase in diagnoses will hit different parts of the world more significantly than others; thus an estimated 90 per cent increase will occur in Europe, 226 per cent in Asia, 345 per cent in Africa and 248 per cent across North and South America.
- More worrying still, out of the 193 member countries of the World Health Organization, only 13 have a national dementia plan – and none of these are in Africa.

The statistics for the UK, provided by Alzheimer's Research UK and the Alzheimer's Society, show the extent to which people in this country contribute to the worldwide dementia figures:

- Currently, 820,000 people in the UK have dementia, meaning that 25 million people know a friend or relative with the condition.
- The number of people in the UK with dementia will at least double by 2050.
- Two-thirds of the people with dementia in the UK are women.
- Dementia costs the economy £23 billion per year, which is more than cancer and heart disease combined; this funding equates to an average of more than £27,000 per person with dementia each year.
- Despite the increased cost of treating dementia, investment in dementia research is almost 12 times lower than for cancer (£50 million versus £590 million per year).

Looking at the Link between Age and Dementia

A clear correlation exists between increasing age and the chances of developing dementia. In fact, fewer than 2 per cent of people are diagnosed under the age of 65. The Alzheimer's Society suggests that the figures can be broken down as follows:

40–64	1 in 1,400
65–69	1 in 100
70–79	1 in 25
80+	1 in 6

The obvious question is whether dementia will become more common as we live longer. Thanks to advances in science, medicine and technology, as a species we're living increasingly longer. Life expectancy until 30,000 years ago is believed to have been less than 30 years, and right up until the 1800s it was common for adults to die by the age of 40. Now the average man in the UK can expect to live for 78.9 years, while a woman can make it to the ripe old age of 82.7.

These figures represent an average, and life expectancy across the UK varies depending on levels of poverty and deprivation. To the same extent, life expectancy in some countries is much lower than in the UK; in Chad, for example, it is, unbelievably, still only 49.5.

Over the next few decades these figures are expected to rise along with the proportion of older people in the population as a whole. According to government figures, currently 10 million people in the UK are over 65 years of age. By 2035, it's estimated that another 5.5 million more elderly people will be resident in the UK, rising to around 19 million by 2050.

A boy born in the UK in 2030 will have a good chance of living until he's 91, and a girl to 95. Given the rising chance of developing dementia with age, it's feared that cases will become far more common as a result of this boom in life expectancy.

Realising that Dementia Doesn't Just Mean Alzheimer's

One of the commonest misconceptions about dementia is that it equals Alzheimer's disease. Alzheimer's disease certainly does equal dementia, but numerous other causes of dementia also exist.

Also consider mild cognitive impairment, which is not yet dementia but not part of the normal ageing process either. For 40 per cent of those who show signs of cognitive impairment, dementia is unfortunately their next step, but for the remainder, their symptoms will either not develop further, or may even be reversible if they are due to depression or the effects of an acute infection.

Considering the 'big four' types of dementia

On safari in Africa, the guides bust a gut to make sure that you get the best chance of glimpsing the so-called 'big five': lions, African elephants, Cape buffalo, leopards and rhinoceros. Dementia can be broken down into the 'big four': Alzheimer's disease, vascular dementia, Lewy body disease and fronto-temporal dementia. Below is a quick field guide to each. (Chapter 3 describes each type of dementia in detail.)

Alzheimer's disease

Alzheimer's disease is the really big one and the most common cause of dementia worldwide. In the UK it's the cause of dementia in 62 per cent of cases, accounting for the symptoms of around 420,000 people.

Alzheimer's is a physical disease that leads to the production of abnormal protein deposits in brain cells, called plaques and tangles. These deposits stop the cells working effectively and eventually kill them off. As the disease progresses, this damage spreads to different parts of the brain, adding to the severity of the symptoms. Symptoms involve changes in memory and other thought processes, alteration of mood and loss of ability to carry out tasks needed for day-to-day living.

Vascular dementia

After Alzheimer's disease, *vascular dementia* is the next most common cause of dementia, affecting about 112,000 people – roughly 17 per cent of the total cases of dementia in the UK. It occurs because of damage to blood vessels around the brain, which in turn limits blood flow and thus oxygen supply to brain cells.

Symptoms are similar to those seen in Alzheimer's disease, but depend on which parts of the brain the reduced blood flow affects. A person who has experienced strokes may also suffer with additional weakness or even paralysis of limbs and speech difficulties.

Because circulation problems become more common as we get older, 10 per cent of people have what's described as *mixed dementia*, where they have Alzheimer's disease alongside vascular dementia, and a mix of symptoms of both.

Lewy body disease

A much rarer sighting, people with *Lewy body disease* make up only 4 per cent of the number of dementia cases – an estimated 25,000 people. Lewy bodies are protein deposits that damage brain cells. They're also found in the brains of people with Parkinson's disease, and as a result an overlap exists in the symptoms of people with these two conditions.

The symptoms of Lewy body dementia are similar to those of Alzheimer's, but sufferers also develop muscle stiffness, tremors and shakiness in their limbs, and slower movement. They can also experience visual hallucinations, commonly seeing animals or people around them that aren't really there.

Fronto-temporal dementia

Fronto-temporal dementia is the smallest of the 'big four', affecting 11,000 people in the UK and representing around 2 per cent of total dementia cases. It's also the most likely of the four types of dementia to be diagnosed in people under the age of 65.

This type of dementia is named because of the areas of the brain that it affects most: the frontal and temporal lobes. These areas of the brain are involved in memory and personality. Thus fronto-temporal dementia shares many of the features of Alzheimer's disease, but has other symptoms, including strange or sexually disinhibited behaviour, lack of empathy, poor personal hygiene, apathy and loss of motivation, increased appetite for sweet or fatty foods, and repetitive and compulsive speech and actions.

Mild cognitive impairment: Dementia lite?

Dementia clearly isn't simply a memory problem, because it affects other thought processes along with mood and the ability to carry out all sorts of everyday tasks. Mild cognitive impairment is often seen as a diagnosis that lies somewhere between full-on dementia and the limitations that occur as a result of a normally ageing brain.

Like dementia, mild cognitive impairment can affect a variety of normal thought processes, but it doesn't impact mood or a person's ability to perform day-to-day functions. And, while it can be a sign of impending dementia for many, especially those with Alzheimer's disease, around 60 per cent of people who develop mild cognitive impairment don't get any worse.

The normally ageing brain

It's no secret that as we get older bits of us start to wear out and don't work quite as well as they once did. Joints become creakier, backs ache, eyesight isn't quite as clear, hair falls out or goes grey, once excitable parts of the body barely raise a smile and memory isn't as sharp as it used to be.

Failing memory was once thought to result simply from a progressive loss of brain cells as we get older, but that's no longer believed to be the case. Research now suggests that unless people have a disease that wipes out their brain cells, they die with the same number that they started life with. And while human brains do shrink in overall size – by about 10 per cent during adulthood – that loss of volume isn't the only culprit behind memory problems.

A combination of factors actually conspire to create the infamous 'senior moments'. These include a reduction in the effectiveness of the communication between nerve cells that whizz information around the brain, an increase of inflammation in brain tissue in response to infection and disease, a reduction in blood supply, and the damage caused by a lifetime's contact with free radical molecules such as oxygen and nitrogen in the atmosphere.

Add these factors to the shrinkage, and you have the recipe for the wear-and-tear type changes we see in the ageing brain as reflexes become slower and people take much longer to finish a crossword than they used to. It's normal, although by no means universal, for people to notice these changes. Some people don't experience even this level of deterioration and are as sharp as tacks well into their 90s (and even beyond).

The abnormally ageing brain

In a person with *mild cognitive impairment*, the symptoms are more significant than those just described for normal ageing. It's not uncommon for people to notice the following:

- ✔ Forgetfulness
- ✔ Difficulty following conversations
- ✔ Declining ability to make sensible decisions
- ✔ Getting lost easily
- ✔ Poor concentration and attention span

The severity of mild cognitive impairment and its progression towards full-on dementia can be charted using the Global Deterioration Scale (GDS) developed by Dr Barry Reisberg in 1982. This score has seven stages:

- ✔ **Stage 1:** No problems identified by doctors or the patient.
- ✔ **Stage 2:** The patient recognises that he has a problem, perhaps with remembering names, but he scores normally on diagnostic tests.
- ✔ **Stage 3:** Subtle problems carrying out thought processes start to affect work and social activities. Tests may well begin to pick up problems (this is mild cognitive impairment).

✔ **Stage 4:** Clear-cut difficulties develop in terms of memory and carrying out tasks such as dealing with finances or travelling. Denial is common. Early dementia has set in.

✔ **Stage 5:** The person needs some assistance but is still quite capable of washing, dressing, eating, going to the toilet and choosing appropriate clothes. Forgetfulness in relation to names and places is becoming more severe.

✔ **Stage 6:** The person is largely unaware of anything that's happened to him in the recent past. He needs help with most of the basic activities of daily living and may need to be looked after in a care home. Incontinence is common.

✔ **Stage 7:** By this stage the person is experiencing severe dementia. He's completely dependent on others for everything, often including mobility. Verbal communication skills are extremely restricted.

Recognising the causes of mild cognitive impairment and taking steps to avoid it

Some cases of mild cognitive impairment are caused by the development of similar protein deposits to those found in Alzheimer's disease. This finding is perhaps not surprising, considering that those people who go on to develop dementia mostly have Alzheimer's disease. Other brain changes noted include worsening blood supply and shrinkage of the part of the brain called the hippocampus, which is involved with memory.

Brain training

A multi-million-pound industry has developed producing specially designed 'brain-training' games and puzzles in response to people's increasing fear of developing dementia.

In 2009, the Alzheimer's Society in the UK teamed up with the BBC science programme *Bang Goes the Theory* to carry out a large-scale experiment looking at the effect of brain training on planning, problem solving and memory. The experiment, 'Brain Test Britain', gathered results from 13,000 people, which were then published in *Nature*, the eminent science journal.

The results clearly showed that while the brain-training exercises made people better at the particularly tasks they were performing, these skills weren't transferred to other brain skills such as memory and planning. And while the research is continuing for the over 60s, the advice for those worried about cognitive impairment is to save money on these specialised products, because they offer no more benefit than do simple crosswords and puzzles.

No specific treatment for mild cognitive impairment exists and, in particular, no evidence suggests that the drugs used to treat Alzheimer's disease are any use. You can gain some mileage, however, by addressing risk factors for poor circulation, by controlling your blood pressure, eating a low-fat and high-fibre diet, quitting smoking, drinking alcohol within the limits of recommended guidelines and taking regular physical exercise.

Some evidence suggests that keeping the brain mentally active by doing word and number puzzles, reading and maintaining stimulating hobbies and social activities can help too.

Considering Copycat Conditions

A whole host of medical conditions can trigger symptoms in people that are very similar to dementia but don't fit the full diagnostic criteria for it. These conditions often cause confusion and can stop people functioning normally in daily life, but they're largely reversible with correct treatment and thus, thankfully, aren't progressive in the same way as dementia is.

When people visit their doctor with symptoms that could mean dementia is setting in, they undergo a number of initial investigations involving blood and urine tests. Such tests are performed to rule out any reversible causes – most frequently, conditions that either affect the brain and nervous system or result from derangements of various bodily hormones. Acute infections can also trigger confusional states, and long-term alcohol abuse can lead to problems with memory (alongside its more commonly seen propensity to render people confused and disorientated).

Neurological causes

Some of the most well-known medical conditions affecting the brain and nerves have symptoms that can mimic some of the features of dementia alongside their own, more specific features. So doctors may want to rule some of these diseases out of their enquiries before coming to a final diagnosis:

- **Parkinson's disease:** This condition does have a genuine overlap with dementia, because people with Parkinson's disease have a higher-than-average risk of also developing dementia. In fact, Parkinson's disease-related dementia accounts for 2 per cent of all cases.

The symptoms of Parkinson's disease-related dementia are very similar to those of Lewy body disease, and researchers think that a link may exist between the two. Thus, alongside problems with cognitive function and movement, people also experience visual hallucinations, mood swings and irritability. Medication to help treat the movement difficulties found in Parkinson's disease, such as tremor and stiffness of muscles, can unfortunately make the symptoms of dementia worse.

✔ **Multiple sclerosis:** In this disease, the outer coating of nerve cells, called myelin, is deficient in some parts of the nervous system, which means that messages carried by the nerves aren't transmitted as well as they should be and may not get through at all. If the nerves affected are in the cortex of the brain, which is where most of the 'clever' functions people perform are carried out, patients can develop cognitive symptoms including forgetfulness and difficulty with problem solving.

✔ **Normal pressure hydrocephalus:** The brain and spinal cord are surrounded by cerebrospinal fluid, which supplies nutrients and acts as a shock absorber to protect the nervous system from damage during trauma. People with hydrocephalus have too much of this fluid, and it begins to damage nerve cells because of the increased pressure. Normal pressure hydrocephalus usually begins to develop in people aged 55 to 60.

The damage that normal pressure hydrocephalus causes in the brain produces symptoms similar to those of dementia, accompanied by difficulties with walking and urinary incontinence. Treatment involves fitting a shunt in the brain to allow the fluid to drain. If the treatment is carried out early in the disease process, the success rate for resolving symptoms is at least 80 per cent.

✔ **Creutzfeldt–Jakob disease (CJD):** This fatal brain disease is, thankfully, rare. It has four types, the most well-known being variant Creutzfeldt–Jakob disease. This version of the disease is believed to be linked to bovine spongiform encephalopathy, better known as BSE or, in tabloid headlines, mad cow disease.

CJD is contagious and is transmitted by an infectious protein called a prion. Once inside the body, prions rapidly destroy brain tissue, leading to death within a year. Symptoms of this awful disease include dementia, unsteadiness, slurring of speech, loss of bladder control and blindness.

✔ **Huntington's disease:** Another of nature's most unpleasant diseases, Huntington's disease is hereditary and is caused by a defect on chromosome 4. If one parent has the disease, a couple's children have a 50:50 chance of inheriting the condition. Symptoms don't develop until middle age, but once they do the disease progresses relentlessly until death. Alongside dementia, sufferers develop jerking movements of their limbs and changes in mood and personality.

Hormonal and nutritional causes

The following conditions are generally not as devastating as the neurological conditions described in the preceding section. Many of the symptoms caused by these conditions are reversible with the correct treatment. Hormonal and nutritional causes of dementia include:

- **Addison's and Cushing's disease:** These conditions, named after the doctors who first discovered them, both affect the levels of a hormone called cortisol. In Addison's not enough cortisol is produced; in Cushing's too much. The knock-on effect of these altered cortisol levels is a corresponding upset in the levels of some of the minerals in the blood stream, most notably sodium and potassium, which leads to confusion. Thankfully, by treating the underlying cause, the confusion is reversible.

- **Diabetes:** One of the most common reasons for doctors seeing people who are acutely confused is that their blood sugar levels are either too low or too high. Neither situation is particularly good for people, but when their blood sugar is adjusted, their confusion quickly fades.

- **Thyroid disease:** Thyroxine is a hormone produced in the thyroid gland, which sits at the front of the neck. In simple terms, this hormone is involved in metabolism within the body: too much and everything in the body is in a rush (the heart races, diarrhoea develops and people become agitated); too little and everything slows down (pulse is slow, people gain weight, skin becomes dry, hair falls out and they can become constipated). Both an under- and over-active thyroid can cause confusion. In both cases, the confusion can again be reversed by treating the underlying cause.

- **Hyperparathyroidism:** The parathyroid glands are pea sized and sit just behind the thyroid gland in the neck. The hormone they produce – parathyroid hormone – is involved in controlling levels of calcium, phosphate and vitamin D. If the gland becomes overactive, levels of calcium in the blood shoot up. Too much calcium can affect personality and consciousness, cause disorientation and, if not corrected quickly enough, coma. Treatment is curative.

- **Vitamin B12 deficiency:** This vitamin, found in fish, poultry, eggs and dairy products, is absorbed in the gut during digestion with the help of a protein called intrinsic factor. Some people either don't make enough of this protein or have a condition that destroys it. As a result, they don't absorb vitamin B12. One of the roles of this vitamin is ensuring healthy nerve function. A lack can cause numbness and tingling in the hands and feet and, if significant, mood changes and poor memory. Treatment by injection of vitamin B12 avoids the problem of lack of stomach absorption and can improve symptoms.

Alcohol-related causes

Indulging in more than the advised levels of society's favourite drug more often than recommended will reveal it to be the poisonous substance it truly is. The effects on the body are wide-ranging and it can wreak havoc on a number of our internal organs, but it's the problems it can cause in the liver and brain that mimic dementia.

- **Cirrhosis:** Liver cells can be damaged by alcohol. The liver can also be affected by viruses such as hepatitis and an autoimmune condition in which the immune system, rather than an infection, attacks the body. Such damage stops the liver working as it should do, which, among other things, leads to the build-up of toxic waste products in the blood. When these toxins build up they can damage brain cells, leading to encephalopathy, which encompasses a collection of symptoms like confusion, poor memory, personality change and inappropriate behaviour. Occasionally, encephalopathy can be reversed by treating the liver damage, but it can prove fatal.

- **Korsakoff's syndrome:** Another condition named after the doctor who discovered it, Korsakoff's syndrome is most often seen in alcoholics in whom high alcohol intake stops the absorption of a B vitamin called thiamine. Thiamine is needed for normal nerve cell function, and insufficient levels commonly cause people to develop memory problems and changes in personality. This condition can be treated by quitting the booze and taking a thiamine supplement.

Infectious causes

Many infections can produce acute confusion, especially in the elderly. This confusion can be caused by the direct effect of viruses or bacteria on the brain, the toxins they produce in the blood stream, or the more general effects of infection on the body, from high temperature to dehydration. The most common infections that can cause confusion – or to give it its more glamorous-sounding, old-fashioned name, delirium – are

- Urinary tract infections such as cystitis (affecting the bladder) and pyelonephritis (affecting the kidneys)
- Chest infections, from bronchitis to full-on pneumonia
- Severe viral infections like influenza
- Infections that directly affect the brain, such as meningitis (which affects the meninges covering the central nervous system) or encephalitis (which affects brain cells)

Prescription medication causes

Although doctors try to follow the age-old dictum 'first do no harm', and medicines are designed to help people get better rather than make them worse, prescribing doesn't always work as planned. We're all different, and in an ideal world all treatment would be bespoke rather than off the peg.

However, we don't live in an ideal world and so, despite doctors' best efforts, their prescriptions may make people, especially older people, feel more unwell than before they collected their pills from the pharmacy. The following medicines can potentially make people acutely confused:

- ✔ Benzodiazepines such as diazepam (valium)
- ✔ Strong painkillers such as tramadol, codeine and morphine
- ✔ Steroids like prednisolone (often used for chronic bronchitis and arthritis)
- ✔ Anticonvulsants such as carbamazepine and phenytoin
- ✔ Anticholinergics, including some hay-fever tablets and medicines used to treat an over-active bladder (such as oxybutynin)

Chapter 2

Spotting the Symptoms

. . . .

. . . .

As doctors, we love to be able to categorise diseases and our ability to do our jobs properly depends on it. It's important to know that set of symptoms A means a patient simply has a nasty dose of the common cold, while set of symptoms B means she's more seriously ill with influenza. Without knowing what someone is up against, we can't advise on treatments or tell her the likely outcome of what she's going through.

In this chapter I look in some detail at the symptoms that show that someone has dementia. And I describe the particular features that allow clinicians to tell people which type of dementia they are suffering from.

Identifying the Early Warning Signs

While dementia affects everyone slightly differently, a few common symptoms can alert you to the fact that it may well be on its way. In the early stages, though, it's important not to panic and see dementia lurking behind every forgetful or confused senior moment, because a failing memory is often simply a normal part of the ageing process. And it is important to bear in mind that there's much more to all types of dementia than simply becoming forgetful.

Differentiating between dementia and a few senior moments

Many things can make all of us absentminded, from simple tiredness and poor concentration to a period of low mood or actual depression. How many of us, busily caught up in an engrossing task or conversation, have forgotten a dental appointment or burnt the dinner?

Only when these symptoms become a regular feature of your behaviour, or that of someone you love, may they be a sign of something more serious. And the symptoms only really become significant when they start to interfere with a person's ability to get on normally with everyday life.

Also, it's rare for memory issues alone to be enough to suggest that dementia is manifesting itself. Problems with finding the right words and confusion over using money or how to follow a favourite recipe are also likely to be evident, alongside changes in mood and loss of confidence in social situations.

Dementia is not just about losing memory.

Knowing what to look out for

Below is a run-down of the top ten most important early symptoms to look out for, as voted for by pretty much every dementia charity website or research article you're likely to come across.

Number 1: Memory problems that affect daily life

Forgetting the odd thing every now and again is perfectly normal as you get older; generally, you remember these things later. In dementia, this doesn't happen: those forgotten things are gone. Unfortunately, you need to remember things such as the following to be able to function normally every day:

- ✔ Important dates and events
- ✔ The route taken on well-travelled journeys
- ✔ Where you've left important paperwork
- ✔ Names and faces of friends, neighbours and work colleagues

Number 2: Difficulty with planning and problem solving

My grandmother could cook a Sunday roast and all the trimmings with her eyes closed – until she started to develop dementia, that is. As the disease took hold, her ability to sort out the timings of meat and vegetables completely deserted her and she'd regularly burn some of the vegetables while undercooking the meat. In the end, Grandpa had to take over the chef's duties or we'd regularly go hungry.

As well as having trouble following recipes, people in the early stages of dementia may also

- ✔ Become confused using a cashpoint card.
- ✔ Lose track of what their bank statement shows.
- ✔ Become confused while trying to put fuel in the car.

Number 3: Problems finding the right word

Most of us will have had the experience of frantically hunting for the right word when chatting to someone or, worse still, when giving a presentation to a group of colleagues. Eventually, the word comes to mind, the panic's over and you stop feeling daft.

In early dementia many people find that words regularly become elusive, leading to difficulty communicating effectively and to huge amounts of frustration. People with early dementia may also substitute the word they're after for something similar, such as a football becoming a kick ball, or a watch becoming a hand clock.

People may also have problems following the thread of other people's conversations, and may therefore become less keen to join in and socialise with others to save themselves embarrassment. Socialising can become a particular problem in noisy environments, or in situations where there are other background conversations going on, because people with dementia will find it harder to focus on the conversation they are supposed to be having.

Number 4: Confusion about time and place

People with early dementia often lose track of time or become muddled about the date. They may also forget where they are or how they got there. As an example, a patient of mine waited in the surgery for ages, expecting to be called in for his consultation with me. Unfortunately, while he did have an appointment at that time, it was across town with his dentist.

Number 5: Poor judgement

Another of the losses that occurs in early dementia is that of good judgement. Normally frugal people may end up spending money on things they don't need, and can be a telesales marketer's dream customer, signing up for all kinds of contract or special offer.

Judgement about appropriate dress may also suffer, with people heading off to the beach wearing a coat, hat and scarf or, conversely, popping to the shops in the pouring rain with only a T-shirt and sandals to protect them from the elements.

Number 6: Visuo-spatial difficulties

The start of dementia can be heralded by increasing clumsiness. As people are robbed of their ability to judge widths and distances, falls and breakages are common, as are bumps (or worse) when parking or driving a car.

Number 7: Misplacing things

While everyone forgets where they've put their keys or mobile phone from time to time, you can usually retrace your steps and eventually find them. This ability to retrace steps is lost in dementia, and coupled with an increasing tendency to leave things in the wrong place as well (slippers in the fridge and so on), important objects increasingly go missing.

Number 8: Changes in mood

My children are teenagers, so rapid mood swings are an extremely common feature of life in my house. One minute a decision I've made means I'm the worst person in the world, and my children feel angry and a bit sorry for themselves; the next (usually when cash has changed hands) I'm a top bloke and they can't think of anyone they'd rather have as a father.

As people grow up into adulthood, these extremes of mood and temperament thankfully tend to be much less evident. But in the early days of dementia this type of fluctuating mood can return, with people often rapidly switching between extremes of sadness, fear and anger. Low mood and full-on depression are also extremely common in dementia. And at times it can be hard to work out whether the symptoms of dementia are causing the depression or vice versa.

Number 9: Loss of initiative

While anyone can become fed up with work, hobbies and even social obligations, this is often a passing phase after a tough day or a bad night's sleep, and you snap out of it. People with dementia may lose the impetus to take part in their usual activities altogether, and repeatedly need prompting about what they should be doing or simply to join in with what friends or family are doing.

Number 10: Personality change

A number of different changes are possible here, and not all people who are developing dementia will change in the same way. In fact, what changes is their normal behaviour, so a reserved and quiet person may become flirty and disinhibited, while the life and soul of many a great party may become withdrawn and reclusive. Common changes include becoming

- Confused
- Suspicious
- Withdrawn

> ✔ Angry
>
> ✔ Sexually disinhibited

As this list demonstrates, the symptoms of dementia are certainly more varied than simply being a bit forgetful. To be diagnosed, someone must show at least two, if not more, of these ten warning signs, which can themselves sometimes be fairly subtle to start with.

As the disease progresses, the symptoms become more obvious, because they become more permanent. The ten symptoms described in this section become part of a person's usual day-to-day life and behaviour, and there's little doubt that the person has developed dementia.

In the rest of this chapter I look in more detail at the symptoms, which can become more severe as time goes on. I split them into symptoms affecting thought processes, mood and the way people function, for ease of explanation, but often a great deal of overlap exists between groups.

For now, I focus on some of the more general symptoms of dementia. People with different types of dementia can develop other symptoms that are particular to their specific diagnosis; for example, Alzheimer's disease or Lewy body disease. Also bear in mind that some people may be lucky enough to develop few of the symptoms I describe, and that the examples in the following section are offered as a guide to what may happen and not what will happen to someone with dementia.

Recognising Thought-Processing Problems

The thought-processing (cognitive) symptoms of dementia are all those of loss. People with dementia will, to one degree or another, lose their memory, their judgement and quite literally their way.

Forgetting

When my uncle George developed Alzheimer's disease, he'd pop to my mum's house round the corner four or five times a day to ask her what she was up to. If he got no reply, he'd post a note through her letterbox that simply said, 'Muriel, where are you?' And all this despite the fact that on his first and no doubt second visit she'd told him exactly what she was up to that day and where she was going.

In contrast, my grandmother, who had vascular dementia, was well aware of everything that was going on each day, but had an awful memory for names and faces. Not only would she mix me up with my brother, but she'd also often call me Bill, which was her son's name.

And the many aspects of forgetting that can occur in dementia go way beyond these two examples from my own family history.

Memory for dates and times

The caricature of a person with dementia is someone who can remember every detail of the Second World War, which she lived through as a child, but can't remember what she had for tea yesterday, or even what day it is. And in a sense, this caricature can be accurate. Dementia tends to involve a loss of short-term memory while many aspects of long-term memory are preserved.

Short-term memory is, in effect, working memory, helping you to function day by day by allowing your brain to remember lists, appointments you need to attend, phone numbers or where you put your door keys. Long-term memory, on the other hand, stores all sorts of information from the past, mingling sights, sounds, smells and the dates of events to give you a rich picture of your life going all the way back to childhood.

In dementia, this loss of short-term memory presents all sorts of problems and can lead to difficulties remembering appointments, important messages and even the day and date, so that the person becomes completely disorientated.

Memories of people and places

Forgetting other people's names and faces is another common problem associated with dementia. These memories are often stored in long-term memory, but when a person experiences problems retrieving these memories, even family members can feel like strangers. This effect on memory can be particularly significant in the workplace, leading to the person with dementia forgetting her boss or important clients.

Forgetting places increases the chance that someone with dementia will easily get lost, even in the most familiar surroundings, and find it very hard to follow the directions of any new route you try to tell her.

Memories of self

When short-term memory malfunctions, it's believed to result in people with dementia losing their sense of self. This mostly affects the present self, and such people may have an intact sense of who they were when they were younger, thanks to their long-term memory.

People with dementia who constantly follow their partners or carers around and keep repeating the same questions may be seeking reassurance and protection from that person to make up for this loss of their own sense of self.

Childhood memories

I vividly remember the first time my dad took me to a football match, on Boxing Day 1974. Not simply because my home team, Portsmouth, beat our arch rivals, Southampton, by four goals to two, but because my long-term memory has stored the associated smell of pipe smoke that in those days wafted around the ground, the sounds of the chanting supporters and the emotional feeling of a 6-year-old doing something grown up with his dad. To this day, every time I get a whiff of pipe smoke I'm transported back to that day, sitting in the North Stand at Fratton Park watching Pompey stuff the Saints.

Getting lost and wandering

When someone's memory for places has ceased to function as it used to, it's very common for her to get lost, even when travelling on extremely familiar routes. In addition, people with dementia tend to wander, which adds to the likelihood that they'll get lost.

Wandering is rarely an aimless activity and would actually be better described as walking with purpose. It is not often obvious to carers why people with dementia sometimes wander, but some suggested reasons include

- ✔ **Continuing with a habit:** People who enjoy walking as either their main means of transport or as a hobby are very likely to continue doing it.

- ✔ **Relieving boredom:** People with dementia often don't have a lot to do, especially as the condition progresses and they withdraw from work and socialising. Going for a walk relieves this boredom and provides a sense of purpose.

- ✔ **Using up energy:** People who were normally quite active and enjoyed exercise may feel restless if they're unable to continue to go out. Going for a walk is a very simple solution.

- ✔ **Being confused:** People with dementia may have an idea they have to be somewhere to do something, but as soon as they've headed off, they become lost and keep wandering, trying to identify familiar landmarks. Sometimes, when confused about time, people with dementia get up in the night thinking it's morning, get dressed and go out. And in severe dementia, they may simply be off to look for someone from their past.

- ✔ **Relieving pain:** People with arthritis stiffen up if they're inactive for long periods, which makes their joints extremely painful. Going for a walk loosens things up and temporarily relieves this pain.

✔ **Searching:** The person with dementia may be off looking for a particular place or person. It may be a former home, or even the house she grew up in. She may be searching for old friends, family members or even long-dead parents.

Progressive lack of judgement

Sensible decision making is key to so many areas of adult life, particularly when it comes to dealing with money, health and the assessment of a multitude of potential risks. Once again, dementia can rob people of this ability, creating potential physical and financial dangers.

Dealing with money

This potential danger can range from people with dementia simply forgetting how to use a cash machine to writing cheques or running up credit card bills for all sorts of charitable causes that they wouldn't normally support or services they don't need and will never use.

I know lots of stories about people who've lost the ability to keep to their overdraft limit or pay off credit card bills on time, and who've been sold unnecessary insurance policies over the phone. In one case, this lack of financial judgement cost the person's employer thousands of pounds.

Awareness of danger

Poor judgement in relation to danger can not only have personal ramifications but also put others at risk. In particular, people with dementia

✔ Have difficulty evaluating the relative risk of situations they find themselves in.

✔ Lose the ability to determine the relative importance of things.

✔ Misjudge environmental conditions and go out unprepared.

✔ Find it hard to think through the logical outcomes of their decisions.

✔ Misjudge the intentions of others.

✔ Overestimate their capabilities.

Put all these elements together and dementia puts people at significant risk of being manipulated or taken advantage of by others, getting robbed or mugged, being a liability behind the wheel of a car or on a bicycle or motorbike, jaywalking (one of my patients was picked up by the police as she wandered along a main road in her nightie) and developing hypothermia as a result of going out in unsuitable clothing and then getting lost.

Observing Emotional Changes

Emotions comprise the next big category of mental functions affected by dementia. In fact, for some people with dementia the term 'emotional roller-coaster' isn't an exaggeration. For families and carers, the emotional changes wrought by dementia can be a huge challenge.

Aggression and agitation

One of the biggest myths about dementia is that everyone who develops it will become angry and aggressive. But while it can happen to some people (studies suggest a range of 30–50 per cent), it's by no means a universal problem and, like anger in other aspects of life, it rarely happens for no reason.

Types of aggression

The aggression expressed by a person with dementia can be both verbal and physical:

- ✔ **Verbal:** Shouting, swearing, screaming, threatening and refusing to comply with a request.
- ✔ **Physical:** Hitting, slapping, biting, scratching, pulling hair and making offensive hand gestures (although these can simply be forms of non-verbal gesturing with no offence intended).

This behaviour can occur in people who were quite aggressive and confrontational before they developed dementia, but can equally arise in people who normally wouldn't hurt a fly. The aggression may just be a phase that the person is going through and may settle with time and appropriate support. And it must be remembered that it may have more to do with the way they are being handled or spoken to, rather than due to an intrinsic pain in their personality.

Reasons behind aggression

Aggressive behaviour can be triggered by a host of physical, psychological and social causes that if adjusted can sometimes alleviate this symptom:

- ✔ **Physical:** Physical aggression can be a direct result of changes in the brain caused by the dementia, or side effects from some of the medication prescribed to treat it. Paranoia, delusions and hallucinations can also prompt protectively aggressive reactions. Equally, however, aggression can be caused by things that would annoy anyone but that generate a more extreme reaction as a result of the disinhibition that can occur due to changes in the brain. These other triggers include noisy surroundings, pain, hunger, thirst and the person simply not getting on with someone.

✔ **Psychological:** A sense of fear and uncertainty is common in dementia, because of the memory and other cognitive problems that it can cause. Feeling frightened and unsure can make people overprotective of themselves, which can lead to anger. Misinterpretation of carers' actions is another common cause of anger. Frustration with their loss of ability to carry out some tasks can also make people irritable, as can, conversely, people being too helpful and not letting patients with dementia do things for themselves.

✔ **Social:** Loneliness, boredom, personality clashes with others and even the well-meaning but poorly performed actions of carers can trigger anger and aggression. If someone poked a sponge on a stick at me while I was in the shower, I'd soon get pretty tetchy with her!

Sexual disinhibition

Sexuality is a normal part of life whether you're young or old, have dementia or don't. People with dementia, however, lose control of the social mechanisms that keep their romantic desires in check at inappropriate moments.

This inability to control sexual impulses can manifest itself very mildly – for example, people are simply more flirtatious or overly familiar with others – but in extreme cases can involve exhibitionism and making unwanted sexual advances. This behaviour is more common in men with dementia than in women, and can involve the following, in descending order of frequency:

✔ Making inappropriate comments

✔ Touching

✔ Fondling

✔ Undressing in public

✔ Making sexual advances

✔ Masturbating in public

The top two on this list are the most common and probably least offensive; the bottom three happen in up to 10 per cent of people with dementia, most commonly as their condition progresses.

Paranoia

People with dementia can develop unfounded fears of being persecuted and can become unnecessarily suspicious of the actions and motives of other people. This paranoia can stem directly from damage to the brain by the process of dementia itself or as a by-product of the confusion that dementia causes. In the latter case, the confusion causes people to misinterpret the actions of others, which they then misconstrue as either negative or outright persecutory. An example here is a husband living in a nursing home believing his wife has maliciously abandoned him, because he can't remember her daily visits or recognise the photographs of her in his room.

Without careful management, this paranoia can provoke unnecessary anxiety, distress and agitation, leading perhaps to more disruptive and aggressive behaviour. Carers can also help reduce it by making sure they are not communicating with the person in oppressive ways or repeatedly restraining her.

Mood swings

Variations in mood are a normal part of life for everyone. On a very basic level, you often feel differently on a Monday morning at the start of a long working week than you do on a Friday, just four mornings later, with the weekend in sight. Your mood goes up before a party, a hot date or after receiving good news, but can swing the other way after learning of a bereavement, when you've been dumped by the hot date or when you experience financial worries.

What's different in dementia is that these mood swings can occur rapidly and without the obvious triggers I've just mentioned. One minute someone may be sitting calmly chatting away to you, and literally the next minute she's pacing the room or crying. The tiniest things can also cause major reactions, with mountains frequently being made out of molehills. This symptom is particularly noticeable if the person concerned has always been quite chilled.

Noting Functional Problems

Alongside the memory problems and emotional changes that happen to someone with dementia, getting in a pickle carrying out practical tasks is the other noticeable development that needs to go hand in hand with the other problems to lead to a diagnosis.

Of course, some of us can make even the simplest practical tasks, from changing a plug to hanging a picture, seem extraordinarily difficult. But in a person with dementia, a combination of changes in the brain can make struggling with many of life's little tasks the rule rather than the exception.

Which shoe on which foot?

As a young man, my uncle was an engineer in the army. In later life he taught often extremely intricate engineering skills to young recruits in the Royal Electrical and Mechanical Engineers. Unfortunately, as an elderly man he developed dementia and became incapable of dressing himself without ending up with something inside out or the buttons done up incorrectly, and even his shoes on the wrong feet.

As a former military man he certainly knew how to dress, and when I was a young army cadet at school he taught me how to shine my boots until I could genuinely see my reflection in their toecaps. But these changes in his attire weren't due to sloppiness because he was running late or had dressed in the dark, which explains most of my wardrobe malfunctions. He got it wrong every time, in different ways, and when his own shoes looked scuffed and unpolished, we knew that something was seriously wrong.

This sort of confusion is extremely common in dementia and is associated with a slowing down of the whole dressing process, because each stage needs to be focused on and is invariably carried out incorrectly. Clothes that were always spotless may start to appear dirty or un-ironed, and the person's appearance may well show a lack of the effort previously put into maintaining it.

This is an example of a problem with what in technical jargon is called *executive function*: putting plans into action. The more steps involved, the more difficult they are to perform.

Kitchen nightmares

While most of us are able to go through the process of preparing a familiar meal without much effort, and can certainly follow a recipe fairly easily, people with dementia start to find this a struggle and would soon have Gordon Ramsey yelling expletives at them if they were cooking in one of his kitchens.

One function of long-term memory is to help you remember how to carry out various common practical procedures, so that you can do them on auto-pilot rather than think each stage through every time. The retrieval of these memories can be impaired in dementia, making the process of changing a plug, riding a bike or whipping up a quick plate of beans on toast more difficult.

Short-term memory problems and difficulties with timing also mean that food can often be burnt, undercooked or left cold in the oven for long enough to grow a layer of mould on top.

Housework becoming a chore

Now I know that not everyone is fastidious when it comes to housework and tidiness. I've visited enough homes as a GP to know that not everyone's floor is clean enough to eat off. (In fact, I've had to sit on my doctor's bag on more than one occasion, because the patient's sofa was teeming with wildlife – Sir David Attenborough could indeed film a mini-series on the contents.)

But a change in the way a formerly house-proud person keeps her home can be another indicator of dementia when coupled with any of the other changes I describe in this chapter. The person may forget to do housework or simply become distracted halfway through, but a dirty home may also be the result of the loss of initiative that features in the top ten early warning signs earlier in this chapter. The houses of the chronically untidy can, of course, simply just become even worse. I remember visiting an old man who was sitting in his armchair surrounded by piles of dirty, mouldy plates and old newspapers, with a bucket in the middle of the room that served as a toilet.

Memory for dummies

A fully functional memory is vital for human existence. That's because without some way of remembering what's happened, every waking moment stands alone as a brand new experience; you have no past and can't plan for the future. Sadly, memory is one of the casualties of the different dementia processes.

Two main types of memory exist: short-term and long-term memory. You also possess an emotional memory, which is completely preserved in dementia, and which I mention at the end of this sidebar.

Short-term memory

Short-term memory is your working memory, which stores information for a short time only (hence its name) before it's either forgotten or transferred to long-term memory for storage, potentially for the rest of your life.

Short-term memory, it's believed, allows people to remember lists of only seven to nine items, for around 30 seconds. Repeating these items over and over in your head can help keep them there, but if you're distracted by something else or the 30 seconds run out, the items are gone.

(continued)

(continued)

Long-term memory

Long-term memory has unlimited capacity and memories can be stored until your dying day. It has two main forms:

✔ **Declarative memory:** This is memory for facts such as bank account or phone numbers, meanings of words, general knowledge and events in your past.

✔ **Procedural memory:** This allows you to remember how to carry out tasks without having to re-learn them each time. It's what makes riding a bike as easy as riding a bike when you haven't done it for a while. And it's what enables us to know how to hold a knife and fork each time we pick them up, or to brush our teeth using the same technique each day.

The development of a long-term memory in the brain involves three crucial steps. If any of these steps don't work, the memory is effectively lost – and that's what can happen in dementia:

✔ Encoding (which ensures that all types of sensory input are in a suitable form for storage)

✔ Storage

✔ Retrieval

Encoding can be thought of as the way in which the nervous system labels a fact, emotion, smell, image or whatever is to be remembered so that it can be stored for further use. It's very similar to the way in which librarians assign specific numbers to books depending on their subject matter so that they can be found easily by someone searching for them among the many bookshelves.

Emotional memory

Emotional memory allows you to recall the really important moments in your life, both good and bad. It stores not only the information about what happened, but an exact memory of how you felt. It means that if you find yourself in a similar situation in future, you'll probably experience those feelings again.

Classic short- and long-term memories are created in a part of the brain called the *hippocampus*, and long-term memories are stored in different parts of the outside of the brain called the *cerebral cortex*. Cells in these areas and those that communicate between them can be damaged in dementia, stopping the encoding, storage and retrieval processes.

In contrast, emotional memory appears to occupy much more primitive parts of the brain, particularly in the brain stem. These areas aren't affected by dementia, meaning that emotional memory can remain intact.

The implication here is that people with dementia can still be troubled by stored memories of negative events, such as the experience of being beaten by a parent as a child. If, because of dementia, a person believes that a long-dead father is still alive, that person may experience some very strong negative emotions. Likewise, an action carried out in the present, such as an injection, that provoked an unhappy response in the past may cause the person with dementia to respond negatively to it. These emotional memories are thought to lead to some of the disturbed and aggressive behaviour seen in people with dementia.

Chapter 3

Looking at the Different Types of Dementia

In This Chapter

▶ Discovering the main types of dementia

▶ Identifying distinguishing symptoms

▶ Taking a brief look at the treatments

Dementia can be very confusing – and not just for the person who has it. This is because no single cause of dementia exists; rather, a number of different diseases may be responsible, each with its own unique signature symptoms. So, rather than being a diagnosis in its own right, *dementia* is actually an umbrella term for the effects that a handful of different neurological conditions can have on the brain and the behaviour of the person who develops them.

In this chapter I look at each of these conditions in detail, focusing on their particular symptoms and causes and the treatments that are being tried to help manage them. I start with the most famous and most common type: Alzheimer's disease.

Understanding Alzheimer's Disease

Alzheimer's disease is the most common form of dementia all over the world, affecting almost 500,000 of the 800,000 people with dementia in the UK. It can affect adults of any age, but becomes more common as people get older.

Alzheimer's disease has a number of stand-out symptoms and unique brain abnormalities that allow doctors to make the diagnosis and therefore point sufferers and their families towards the best forms of treatment as quickly as possible.

Taking a quick look at the history of the disease

The history books say that this type of dementia was first discovered in 1910, by the man whose name the condition bears: Dr Alois Alzheimer. But many historians have since pointed out that the truth is not quite so straightforward, and that

- ✔ The condition was actually already recognised in the 1800s.

- ✔ The case history that Dr Alzheimer described didn't fit the exact criteria for what is now known as Alzheimer's disease.

- ✔ It was the doctor's colleague, the psychiatrist Dr Emil Kraepelin, who named the disease Alzheimer's disease.

Dr Alzheimer's patient was a 51-year-old woman, Auguste D, who was an inpatient in a state-run psychiatric hospital in the German city of Frankfurt. She'd been admitted in 1901 not only for problems with her memory and thought processes but also because she was paranoid, quite aggressive and was hearing voices. When she died in April 1906, her brain was sent for post-mortem examination, and Alzheimer presented the findings at a scientific meeting the following year. It was not until three years later, though, that Kraepelin labelled her condition Alzheimer's disease.

Dementia in the 19th century

The term 'dementia' was already in use as a diagnosis during Alois Alzheimer's time to describe any condition in which people demonstrated problems with mental or social functioning, whether or not the condition was temporary and reversible, and regardless of their age.

Over time the diagnosis became more finely tuned and ended up, as it is now, being applied to conditions that are irreversible and lead to gradual deterioration in someone's memory, thought processes and ability to carry out the ordinary activities of daily living, such as shopping, cooking, cleaning and washing.

The patient in question, though, demonstrated other symptoms such as hallucinations and paranoid ideas that no longer fit into the current criteria for diagnosing Alzheimer's disease. So the patient was far from being a classic case of the condition she was used to describe.

A unique disease

The post-mortem findings on Auguste D's brain were the clincher that enabled doctors to announce that this was a brand new and identifiable disease in its own right. In Auguste D's brain cells they found

- Protein plaques
- Neurofibrillary tangles

These cells are both formed by abnormal folding of proteins.

But again, Alzheimer wasn't the first to find these sorts of changes in the brains of people who had dementia. A Dr Fuller in the USA had identified the tangles five months before Alzheimer reported on his post-mortem, and in the late 1880s scientists in Europe had identified protein plaques.

What's in a name?

The disease now known as Alzheimer's disease was far from being a new discovery when it was described. In fact, historians think that Kraepelin made his announcement simply because the academic department at his university needed a funding boost and this 'discovery' brought it much-needed publicity.

Nevertheless, the name has stuck, and regardless of its slightly dodgy origins, I now go on to look at what doctors mean when they diagnose someone as having Alzheimer's disease in the 21st century.

Spotting the main symptoms

Despite the controversial nature of the condition's beginnings, doctors now have a very clear-cut set of symptoms that they use to identify whether someone has developed Alzheimer's disease.

The symptoms often develop slowly, with researchers believing that from the start of the changes that Alzheimer's causes in the brain it may take as long as 15 years to produce a full textbook set of symptoms.

While a fair amount of overlap in symptoms exists between Alzheimer's disease and the other different types of dementia, each type has its own stand-alone features. These symptoms affect – to a greater or lesser extent, depending on the type of dementia – three main types of brain activity and social functioning:

- Memory and thought processes
- Mood and emotions
- Activities of everyday living

Memory and thought processes

The effects on memory and thought processes are the symptoms that most people think of when they think about dementia. My patients often come to see me because they think that they're either losing their memory or, if they're being unkind to themselves, losing their marbles. Whatever they say, they always come with a real sense that something somewhere inside their heads has been lost.

And it's not just memory that can go missing: the marbles certainly shouldn't be left out either, because far more than just the ability to recall things goes awry in Alzheimer's disease.

Memory

Two main types of memory exist: short-term and long-term memory (which Chapter 2 covers in detail). But, for now, the basics of each are as follows:

- ✔ *Short-term memory:* This is what's often called working memory, because it allows you to remember things like telephone numbers and shopping lists, conversations you've recently had and what was for breakfast. It has limited capacity, however, so facts don't stay there for long before they're either forgotten or transferred to long-term memory.

- ✔ *Long-term memory:* This has unlimited capacity and allows you to remember things for the rest of your life. Long-term memory retains not only facts, such as who won the FA Cup in 1975 (West Ham United, beating Fulham 1–0), but also sights, smells and sounds from the past (the smell of school dinners, for example, or your nan's favourite perfume). It also allows you to remember how to perform tasks such as tying your shoelaces and riding a bike.

Memory loss

In Alzheimer's disease, short-term memory tends to be lost first. This means that people will often get to the shops and forget what they went there for; forget the names of family and friends, even if they see them regularly or have known them for years; and keep losing things that they may have just put down but can't remember where.

Long-term memories, however, often remain completely intact, with sufferers seemingly reverting to living in the past. As the disease progresses, people may increasingly appear to live in the world they inhabited as children. They often think of themselves as being much younger than they are, and talk as if long-dead parents are still alive.

Memories of conversations will also be lost and lead to the person repeatedly asking the same questions that have already been answered, or ringing family and friends over and over again to repeat a discussion. They might also repeatedly tell you the same stories or discuss strong memories because these are things they feel confident or strongly about.

Loss of other mental abilities

As memory declines, other thought processes follow suit. A number of previously simple tasks and activities can become unbelievably tricky and frustrating for the person with Alzheimer's disease. The effects include

- ✔ Poor memory for places, which can lead people to become lost easily, even in what were once familiar neighbourhoods.

- ✔ Wandering (walking with purpose), which can develop once people start to lose their bearings when out and about, or if they head off to do something and forget what it was midway through their journey. Leaving the front door unlocked in their haste to get going somewhere isn't uncommon either.

- ✔ Items of clothing and household equipment frequently becoming lost, because they've been stored in the wrong place, such as slippers in the fridge or milk bottles in the oven.

- ✔ Judgement becomes severely impaired, so that people with Alzheimer's disease may put on clothes unsuitable for current weather conditions, and may wrap up in jumpers and scarves on a warm midsummer's day, or go out in the rain in just a blouse. Judgement about money and finances will also be affected, leading not only to people buying things they don't need but also to them having trouble recognising the correct coins and notes to pay for them with.

Mood and emotions

The next category of symptoms features changes in mood and emotions. These changes may be the first that people notice – 'Dad's just not himself any more' – but can be mimicked by other conditions such as depression or anxiety, and so can easily be missed.

Mood changes

Mood changes can be long term, with previously happy-go-lucky people becoming noticeably down and depressed and not being able to shake out of it. But mood changes can also be temporary, with a swing from laughter to tears happening quickly.

Emotional changes

Irritability (and perhaps even full-on aggression) is one of the symptoms that many people associate with Alzheimer's disease. And it certainly can be a feature of the condition. (It can also be an emotion that springs from fear, threat or frustration, rather than occurring for its own sake – see Chapter 9.)

Irritability is by no means a universal symptom, however, and some people remain very mild and placid when they develop this type of dementia. Other alterations that may occur in someone's emotions include

✔ Paranoid and suspicious behaviour in relation to family members or neighbours. Sufferers believing that people are spying on them or stealing possessions from them is common.

✔ Impatience with people and ignorance of the very British convention of queuing because of disinhibition in these circumstances.

✔ Sexually disinhibited speech or behaviour and over-familiarity with strangers.

✔ Inappropriate laughter or tears.

The penultimate emotional change was a big feature of my grandmother's dementia. She never missed an opportunity to flash a suspender belt in public or whip out her ample chest for her medical student grandson to examine with his stethoscope. Thankfully, she kept her bra on, or her grandson may have given up his studies there and then and wouldn't be writing this book.

Activities of daily living

This term describes the tasks that people carry out every day, such as preparing meals, taking a bath and shopping for groceries. These activities are things you usually take for granted and perform so often that you could do them with your eyes closed.

In the early stages of Alzheimer's disease, however, people can find these simple tasks increasingly difficult. As the disease progresses, it can unfortunately reach the stage where some people have to be fed and have the most basic procedures, like wiping their bottoms, done for them by others. Preparing meals, washing, cleaning, doing the laundry and sorting household bills can all become quite a struggle.

Acknowledging the risk factors

The jury's still out on a cause for Alzheimer's disease. A single trigger is unlikely to exist – no special virus or particular noxious chemical in the water; rather, a number of different factors in a person's genetic make-up, lifestyle and environment probably gang up on him to cause the disease to develop. Chapter 4 covers the causes of Alzheimer's disease in a lot more detail, but below is a quick, whistle-stop tour of the main culprits.

Genetics

A fair amount of evidence suggests that genes can play a part in the development of Alzheimer's disease. The genetic link varies depending on whether a person has early-onset Alzheimer's, which affects people aged between 30 and 60, or the far more common late-onset Alzheimer's, which strikes from the age of 60 onwards.

Early onset

This is the rare form of the disease and accounts for 5 per cent of all cases of Alzheimer's. It seems to be inherited from people's parents as a result of mutations in one of a number of genes when they're passed on. The list of the genes responsible continues to grow in response to ongoing research.

Late onset

In people over the age of 60 with Alzheimer's, one of the genetic culprits is thought to be the gene for apolipoprotein E (APOE), although probably another 20 genes may also play a part. APOE is involved in breaking down a type of protein called beta amyloid inside brain cells. A problem with the gene means a problem producing APOE, and a person without it is at risk of building up beta amyloid. This build-up, which is a hallmark in Alzheimer's disease, damages brain cells.

I look at genetics in more detail in Chapter 4.

Lifestyle factors

A wealth of evidence shows that decline in memory and other thought processes can be brought on by reductions in blood supply to brain cells. This in turn is triggered by damage to blood vessels, which is caused by the unholy trinity of

- ✔ Smoking
- ✔ Poor diet
- ✔ Lack of exercise

Add in obesity, large quantities of alcohol, diabetes and uncontrolled high blood pressure and you have the ingredients for Alzheimer's disease.

Lack of social contact is also thought to be a risk factor for the disease, with isolation and mental inactivity both being contributory factors.

The environment

For once, this environmental message isn't about global warming, the destruction of the rainforests or acid rain (although none of them should be ignored in the grand scheme of things). Where Alzheimer's is concerned, scientists have suggested that our ingestion of pesticides such as DDT and certain nitrogen-containing fertilisers used in agriculture could be increasing our risk of developing the disease.

The links aren't proven yet, but the environment could well be one more piece of the jigsaw.

Working through the tests

The results of no single test will tell a doctor that someone has Alzheimer's disease; no blood test, scan or questionnaire alone is sufficient to pinpoint the diagnosis. This situation is a pain because without investigatory certainty people showing the symptoms of dementia will to an extent remain somewhat of a medical mystery.

Thankfully, a few different tests do exist that when put together can point towards a diagnosis. Diagnosis is a bit like assembling a jigsaw puzzle: the picture generally becomes clearer bit by bit. Although at times the picture, and therefore the diagnosis, can change.

Blood tests

Although no blood test exists to identify Alzheimer's disease, a doctor nevertheless will send a person for a number of blood tests in order to rule out a handful of conditions that can cause dementia-like symptoms. These include tests for

- Anaemia
- Thyroid gland dysfunction
- Diabetes
- Electrolyte (sodium and potassium) and calcium imbalance
- Vitamin deficiencies (particularly vitamin B12 and folic acid)

Urine test

Simple urinary-tract infections, such as cystitis, can cause older people to become quite dramatically confused. And while this confusion generally won't be longstanding (except in a few cases when it can last for six months after the infection has cleared), as it is in dementia, making sure that a urinary infection isn't all that's wrong with someone before subjecting him to some of the more high-tech, detailed tests is definitely worthwhile.

Scans

Brain scans can often prove to be the final piece of the diagnostic jigsaw in Alzheimer's disease. Three main types of scan are used, the choice of which is guided by a person's symptoms.

CT scan

Computerised tomography (CT) scans are most commonly used. They involve laying someone in what looks like a large doughnut and then passing x-ray beams, painlessly, through his brain. The pattern of these rays is interpreted by a computer, which builds up a picture of the brain that can then be examined in slices from top to bottom.

MRI scan

Magnetic resonance imaging (MRI) scans use magnetic fields and radio waves rather than x-rays to make pictures of the brain. MRI scans are also analysed in slices through the various levels of the brain. MRI scans are particularly good at picking up problems with blood vessels deep within the brain.

SPECT

Single-photon emission computerised tomography (SPECT) scans use a particular type of radioactive ray called a gamma ray to build up a three-dimensional picture of the brain. This type of scan can be used to look at metabolism, in particular regions of the brain, and pick up the characteristic abnormalities in metabolism seen in Alzheimer's disease, for which it is over 70 per cent sensitive.

SPECT scans, however, are expensive and not always available. Hence they're generally used only if diagnosis is still unclear using the other scanning techniques, or for a fee in a private hospital.

In a person with Alzheimer's disease, the scans can show a generalised reduction in brain volume, particularly in the region of the temporal lobe called the hippocampus, which is involved in the processes of memory.

DAT Scans

DopAmine Transporters (DAT) scans let clinicians know how much dopamine a person has in his brain. DAT scans involve the injection of radioactive chemicals into the blood stream. These attach to nerve cells in the brain that use the neurotransmitter dopamine to transmit signals.

More commonly used to help diagnose Parkinson's disease, in which there is a loss of dopamine, they can also be used to differentiate between Lewy body disease and Alzheimer's disease.

Cognitive tests

Last but by no means least in diagnosing Alzheimer's disease are the cognitive tests. These are administered by specialist nurses, doctors and psychologists with the aim of pinpointing exactly which areas of memory and thought processing a person is having trouble with.

Different patterns of results in these cognitive tests are demonstrated by the main types of dementia, which allows the diagnosis to become yet clearer.

Looking at treatment options

No cure for Alzheimer's disease exists, but four different drugs can currently be used to slow its progression and improve some of the cognitive symptoms. These drugs stabilise symptoms, with patients often reporting improvements in the first six months of taking them. The available drugs are

- ✔ Donepezil
- ✔ Galantamine
- ✔ Rivastigmine
- ✔ Memantine

I look at these in detail in Chapter 7.

Other behavioural and psychological treatments can help manage the tricky symptoms that may develop as the disease progresses.

Being realistic about the outlook

Alzheimer's disease is as yet incurable, and so the symptoms get progressively worse over time. That time can, however, vary dramatically between people with the condition: life expectancy after diagnosis can range from 5 to 20 years. Life expectancy obviously depends on the severity of the Alzheimer's disease and the type and level of care available.

Explaining Vascular Dementia

Vascular dementia is the second most common type of dementia, accounting for around 20 per cent of all cases of dementia diagnosed in Europe. In the UK, at least 100,000 people have vascular dementia.

Experiencing problems with circulation

A reduction in blood flow to brain cells is the main problem in vascular dementia. Insufficient blood flow means that inadequate oxygen is supplied to these brain cells, which will begin to die as a result. And the death of large numbers of brain cells can lead to dementia.

Identifying which circulatory problems are responsible

The triggers for a reduction in blood flow can be the result of damage to blood vessels around the brain itself or the body's circulation in general. These include

- Strokes
- Transient ischaemic attacks (TIAs; mini strokes that settle after 24 hours)
- General furring-up of the arteries (atherosclerosis)
- Haemorrhage
- Heart failure

Binswanger's disease

Binswanger's disease is a specific type of vascular dementia that's caused by damage to small blood vessels deep within the subcortical regions of the brain. In contrast, the more common-or-garden type of vascular disease affects areas of the cortex.

The disease causes damage to blood vessels that's colloquially termed *hardening of the arteries*. It again reduces blood flow to brain cells, causing them to die. It tends to develop in people in their 50s and 60s, and gets progressively worse with age.

Spotting the symptoms

Symptoms of vascular dementia are similar to those of Alzheimer's disease, although they may also be accompanied by other neurological symptoms, such as one-sided limb weakness or other signs that the person has experienced strokes. As a result of this link to strokes and transient ischaemic attacks (TIAs), the progression of vascular dementia has traditionally been described as proceeding in a stepwise fashion: new strokes or episodes of worsening blood flow in the brain lead to a further deterioration in cognitive symptoms.

This stepwise process doesn't happen in all patients with vascular dementia, some of whom will show the steady progression of their dementia in the way that occurs in Alzheimer's disease. This is often particularly the case in people with Binswanger's disease.

The other symptoms to look out for are

- Decline in cognitive function and worsening memory
- Unsteadiness when walking
- Personality change, often featuring aggression

- Depression
- Visual and auditory hallucinations (seeing and hearing things that aren't there)
- Frequent urge to pass urine, sometimes associated with incontinence

Acknowledging the risk factors

The list of risk factors for vascular dementia reads a bit like a *Who's Who* of risk factors for all kinds of blood vessel damage. Here goes:

- Increasing age
- High blood pressure – public enemy number one for blood vessels
- Heart disease, especially heart attacks, angina, abnormally functioning heart valves (which can develop tiny clots that whizz off to the brain) and a type of irregular heartbeat called atrial fibrillation
- Hardening of blood vessels, called atherosclerosis
- Diabetes, particularly if it's not well controlled
- Smoking (just don't do it!)
- Genetic problems, specifically an inherited condition known as CADASIL because its full name (cerebral autosomal dominant arteriopathy with subcortical infarcts and leukoencephalopathy) is a bit of a mouthful

---

CADASIL

CADASIL is, thankfully, a rare condition. It's caused by a gene abnormality on chromosome 19. It affects around 1 in 200,000 people and is found equally in men and women. The condition is passed from affected parents to their children, who have a 50 per cent chance of inheriting the gene.

The first symptoms usually develop in patients in their 20s. These symptoms are generally frequent episodes of migraine headaches that are preceded by an aura, which might manifest itself as zig-zagging lines in the field of vision of one eye, or dizziness, sensitivity to light or ringing in the ears.

In their 30s, people with CADASIL can begin to have strokes and TIAs, and may also start to develop the symptoms of dementia. These symptoms become worse over the following 20 years and most sufferers die, very prematurely, in their 50s.

CADASIL can be picked up on brain scans, but even with an early diagnosis no cure exists and the only treatments available are aimed at helping to relieve the symptoms.

Working through the tests

The initial procedure for diagnosing vascular dementia is the same as for Alzheimer's disease, including

- ✔ A full medical history looking for a history of strokes or TIAs, plus any urinary or mobility issues
- ✔ A clinical examination, in which blood pressure and cardiac tests may be particularly useful, together with a neurological check if the person has had a stroke in the past
- ✔ Baseline blood and urine tests
- ✔ Cognitive tests for 'memory testing'

 In diagnosing vascular dementia, however, the scans are most likely to be particularly helpful. Brain scans such as CT or MRI, described in relation to Alzheimer's disease earlier in this chapter, are used to find evidence of strokes, TIAs and blood vessel abnormalities.

If these scans show signs of vascular changes, the doctor may also want to carry out other specific scans of the patient's circulation. These scans will look at blood vessels in the neck, using a type of ultrasound scanner to look at blood flow (carotid artery Doppler scans) and blood flow through the heart (echocardiogram). Problems in both of these areas may put a person more at risk of further strokes or TIAs and can possibly be treated.

Looking at treatment options

Unfortunately, as with Alzheimer's, vascular dementia is a progressive and untreatable disease. But by achieving better control of the risk factors for the condition, deterioration can be slowed down and possibly halted, and further strokes and TIAs prevented. Lifestyle advice will be offered, and a variety of different medications prescribed.

The advice to a person with vascular dementia is as follows:

- ✔ If you smoke, stop smoking.
- ✔ If you eat a high-fat, low-fibre diet, try to switch it around to a low-fat, high-fibre one.
- ✔ Cut down on alcohol.
- ✔ Do some exercise if your general physical condition allows it.

Medication will be aimed at

- ✔ Optimising blood pressure control, so that your blood pressure is as good as it will get.
- ✔ Making sure your cholesterol level is within the recommended range.
- ✔ Treating diabetes, if you have it, to ensure the best possible blood sugar control.
- ✔ Thinning the blood to prevent further strokes or TIAs.

Finally, the patient may be prescribed drugs for Alzheimer's disease (donepezil, galantamine, rivastigmine or memantine) to see whether they help with the cognitive symptoms of vascular dementia, but only if it's felt that the person has a mixture of the two conditions.

Being realistic about the outlook

The outlook for people with vascular dementia is unpredictable. But statistics suggest that approximately one-third of people with this diagnosis will die as a direct result of its complications, while a further one-third will die from strokes as a result of their cerebrovascular disease. Lifespan will be reduced for all types of vascular dementia.

Getting to Grips with Mixed Dementia

Mixed dementia is the third most common form of dementia, and it becomes increasingly common with advancing age.

Having two types of dementia at once

As the name suggests, people with mixed dementia have more than one type of dementia process co-existing in their brains, although this does not mean that they have a double dose. The most common combination is Alzheimer's disease plus vascular dementia, but Alzheimer's can also be combined with Lewy body disease. And reports also exist of people having Alzheimer's disease plus vascular dementia plus Lewy body disease – but fortunately these cases are rarer.

Despite all the tests that doctors can throw at dementia to try to work out an exact diagnosis, it's still not 100 per cent possible to tease the symptoms apart and get a completely accurate diagnosis for everyone. As a result, probably far more people have mixed dementia than the number that doctors are at present able to give that diagnosis to.

Spotting the symptoms

Identifying the symptoms is a bit tricky because it depends on which dementias are mixed together. And the situation isn't as straightforward as thinking that because a person has dementia type A mixed with dementia type B, symptoms of both will be visible in equal measure.

 Consider a slightly left-field analogy to describe dementia. If a plate of food represents the sum of your symptoms, it won't resemble a serving of Sunday roast with the meat and two veg arranged next to each other so you can pick out the individual flavours. Instead, the food will be more like a stew, where the tastes of the meat, herbs and vegetables are blended and so less distinctive.

The symptoms themselves are mainly those recognisable in Alzheimer's disease and vascular dementia (and described in the earlier sections of this chapter) and therefore include the associated symptoms of heart disease, strokes or TIAs. Different people will exhibit the symptoms of each to different extents.

Acknowledging the risk factors

Mixed dementia is caused by a mixture of pathological processes in the brain, but most commonly those of Alzheimer's disease, together with conditions affecting the circulation, such as furring-up of the arteries or strokes.

Working through the tests

When people first go to see their doctor, they're put through the same basic tests that the section on Alzheimer's covers, to make sure that dementia is what they're suffering from, and then to tease out which type. A person is likely to have a mishmash of symptoms, which will lead to the diagnosis of mixed dementia.

Brain scans may also reveal features of both Alzheimer's disease and vascular dementia, showing evidence of

- ✔ A general loss of brain cells, but particularly in the temporal lobe in the area of the hippocampus
- ✔ Evidence of strokes, TIAs or general hardening of the arteries

Looking at treatment options

Unfortunately, as with its component parts, no cure exists for mixed dementia. But it does seem to respond to some of the drugs used to treat Alzheimer's disease, such as donepezil, galantamine and rivastigmine.

And as with people with vascular dementia, someone with mixed dementia benefits from adequate treatment to

- ✔ Control blood pressure.
- ✔ Lower cholesterol.
- ✔ Prevent any further strokes, heart attacks or TIAs.

Being realistic about the outlook

The outlook for mixed dementia is much the same as that for vascular disease: that is, lifespan is reduced for all sufferers.

Analysing Fronto-Temporal Dementia

Fronto-temporal dementia (FTD) is a very specific type of dementia that only affects certain parts of the brain, giving it both its name and symptom pattern. It's probably the rarest of the main types of dementia and tends to run in families.

Recognising why it's different

This type of dementia can start earlier than the others and is most often diagnosed under the age of 65, often in people as young as 45 years old. FTD is also unusual because it's very selective for only two areas of the brain: the frontal lobes (at the front) and the temporal lobes (at the sides).

Fronto-temporal dementia was first identified as a unique condition in 1892 by psychiatrist Arnold Pick. For many years, it understandably went by the name Pick's disease.

Spotting the symptoms

Three variants of this condition exist, each with its own idiosyncratic symptoms depending on which parts of the brain are particularly affected.

Behavioural variant FTD

If you have this type of FTD, you can develop the following symptoms:

- Loss of inhibition, causing socially inappropriate and often tactless behaviour
- Loss of interest in people and things (but you exhibit no features of depression)
- Loss of sympathy and empathy
- Repetitive and compulsive behaviours such as hoarding and obsession with timekeeping
- Binging on junk foods, cigarettes and alcohol; increased sweet tooth

Unlike other types of dementia, however, memory isn't a major issue.

Language variants of FTD

Two variants of FTD involve disruption of normal language:

- **Progressive non-fluent aphasia:** In this variant the sufferer may have slow, hesitant speech, with frequent stuttering and a tendency to mis-pronounce words. Grammar can be affected, so that people leave out connecting words such as 'the' and 'to' from sentences.
- **Semantic FTD:** Here, speech is fluent but a person may have problems finding the right words for objects or names for people. This leads people to use a generic word like 'animal' because 'tiger' won't come to mind.

Overlapping syndromes

About 20 per cent of people with FTD also develop a muscular disorder to go with it, such as motor neurone disease or progressive supranuclear palsy. Together with the symptoms of dementia and the particular type of FTD, a person may thus also experience muscle twitching and weakness in various parts of the body.

Acknowledging the risk factors

A big genetic component to FTD exists; in fact, 10 to 20 per cent of people who develop this disease inherit it from their parents. The damage to the cells is caused by abnormal proteins forming in brain cells, which seems to destroy them.

Working through the tests

At the risk of sounding repetitive, the initial stages of investigation are the same as for all other types of dementia, and the doctor looks for the specific symptoms described in the earlier sections of this chapter. The patient's age and any family history will lead the doctor to consider FTD.

Brain scans may well show reduced brain tissue in the frontal and temporal lobes, and a SPECT scan can specifically show reduced levels of brain activity in these areas too. If the patient has a strong family history of this disease, genetic tests might also prove helpful in reaching the diagnosis.

Looking at treatment options

As with all the other types of dementia, the medical profession has yet to come up with an effective treatment to either cure FTD or to even slow its progress and the drugs used to treat Alzheimer's disease can actually make things worse. Most treatments are aimed at reducing the severity of symptoms and their impact on others. Almost exclusively behavioural treatments will be recommended for FTD; Chapter 8 covers these in detail.

Being realistic about the outlook

The FTD variants of dementia all become steadily worse over time, producing a disabling combination of declining social, cognitive and neurological functions. This situation inevitably means that people with FTD will need long-term nursing-home care. The length of this care is variable: some people, especially those with motor neurone disease, die within five years of diagnosis, and others can survive with the disease for up to ten years.

Discovering Dementia with Lewy Bodies

Dementia with Lewy bodies (DLB), which affects around 100,000 people in the UK, is unique in terms of the brain changes that occur and some of the symptoms that result.

Recognising why it's different

Having just billed DLB as being unique, it's now only fair to briefly state why.

Lewy bodies

The crucial difference in the brain of someone with Lewy body disease is the presence of the Lewy bodies themselves. In 1912, while working on the brains of people who in life had experienced symptoms of dementia, Frederick Lewy, after whom the bodies are named, noted abnormal spherical protein deposits in the midbrain and cortex.

Symptoms affecting movement

Lewy bodies are also found in the brains of people with Parkinson's disease, and so people with this type of dementia often have a number of symptoms that affect their movement.

Spotting the symptoms

People with DLB not only have symptoms of dementia in common with all the other dementias I describe in this chapter, but they also have some symptoms in common with people who have Parkinson's disease. The diagnosis of DLB depends on the presence of two out of three core symptoms, plus or minus any of a number of supportive symptoms.

Core symptoms

The core symptoms the doctor looks for are

- **Fluctuating consciousness:** People with DLB experience large swings in levels of confusion, so that on some days the confusion is extreme and they're unable to function, and on others they can follow the plot of a film or play a game of cards pretty decently. These fluctuations can also happen minute by minute or hour by hour.

- **Visual hallucinations:** Around two-thirds of people with DLB experience *visual hallucinations* (seeing things that aren't really there but are so vivid that they seem real). These can be quite pleasant for some people, but frightening hallucinations can be particularly distressing.

- **Spontaneous Parkinsonism:** *Spontaneous Parkinsonism* produces the usual symptoms of Parkinson's disease, such as muscle stiffness, slow movement, tremors, shakiness and loss of facial expression.

Supporting symptoms

Together with the core symptoms of DLB, a person may experience

- Fainting
- Falls
- Problems swallowing

- ✔ Incontinence
- ✔ Delusions
- ✔ Depression
- ✔ Acting out dreams, sometimes violently, as a result of a specific problem called rapid eye movement (REM) sleep disorder

Acknowledging the risk factors

No one yet knows what causes DLB. It doesn't seem to run in families and no common gene abnormalities have been found to explain it.

Working through the tests

The diagnosis of DLB depends largely on the medical history of dementia plus the core and supporting symptoms listed in the 'Spotting the symptoms' section. No scan can prove that a person has DLB, but scans are still useful because they'll at least rule out other causes such as Alzheimer's disease and vascular dementia.

Looking at treatment options

Sadly, no specific treatment for DLB exists, although some of the Alzheimer's disease medications can help to reduce the symptoms for a few months and slow their deterioration (rivastigmine, for example, can ease hallucinations). Other medication can be used to help alleviate its symptoms:

- ✔ Clonazepam can help with REM sleep disorder.
- ✔ Selective serotonin reuptake inhibitor (SSRI) antidepressants such as Prozac can help the depression that's a common feature of DLB.

Although people with DLB can experience psychotic symptoms, such as delusions and hallucinations, they're very sensitive to the effects of the anti-psychotic drugs that are usually used to treat them, which can cause severe side effects.

Being realistic about the outlook

DLB is incurable and has a similar outlook to Alzheimer's disease.

Chapter 4

Considering Causes and Risk Factors

*P*revention, everyone is told, is better than cure. And with dementia, for which no cure exists and the symptoms are so devastatingly awful, surely anything is worth trying in order to keep the disease at bay. Unfortunately, no one single thing that you can do or not do prevents dementia. The situation isn't as simple as with some other conditions where you can say 'wash your hands after going to the toilet and you'll avoid getting diarrhoea' or 'don't eat pie and chips every day and you won't become obese' or 'have your vaccinations when you're younger and you won't get mumps'.

Doctors can't put their fingers on a single trigger for dementia, which is perhaps not surprising given that it manifests itself in many different ways. Thankfully, however, some scientific evidence suggests that changing diet and lifestyle – keeping mentally and physically active – can help you avoid developing dementia.

This chapter looks at the different risk factors, from genes to environmental pollutants, from lack of exercise to a 20-a-day smoking habit. First, though, it offers a quick overview of how your brain and memory work when they're not affected by disease, to help you get a better understanding of what goes wrong in dementia and how you can help yourself to try to avoid it.

Taking a Quick Look Under the Bonnet (Barnet)

Computers are now ubiquitous. Pretty much everyone, regardless of their age – from nursery school children to silver surfers – has at least one electronic gadget. Mobile phones, tablets, laptops and gaming consoles – everyone's familiar with machines containing microchips that are seemingly so clever they can almost think for themselves. Maybe one day they will.

Thus looking inside the skull at the human brain (or at least a picture of it) and discovering that it contains no shiny components or intricate circuitry can be a shock. And the confusion is compounded by the fact that, unlike other organs in the body, the brain doesn't look like what it does. The heart, for example, is unmistakably a pump, the long, tubular guts are clearly designed to have something passing through them, and the lungs, with their tiny airspaces, are obviously used for breathing. Thankfully, the strange, waxy-looking organ inside your head is a lot cleverer than it looks. In fact, it's the most technically clever object in the whole of the known universe.

At this moment, for example, my brain is controlling my hands as they tap the keyboard; my eyes are sending it images of the words as they form on the screen; I can hear music from my iPod and sense the presence of my budgerigar, Frank, as he flaps around the room behind me. As well as processing all that information, my brain is also thinking of the next words to write, composing sentences with them and planning the paragraphs that they'll eventually construct. And all the while it's controlling my breathing, heart rate, balance and everything else needed to keep me alive and conscious, while simultaneously storing and recalling memories. And it does all this, and so much more, 24 hours a day without breaking a sweat.

Considering normal brain structure and function

This is obviously a bit of an ambitious title for a small section in a book, because you could fill whole libraries with tomes and research papers on which bits of the brain are where, the routes through which they communicate with each other and the chemical processes involved, and still not have all the answers. The pathways controlling muscle movement are complicated enough, let alone the ones scientists think determine personality and stimulate feelings such as love.

But you have to start somewhere, so here's a rough outline of the brain's anatomy and the method by which messages whizz around it, allowing you to do all the clever physical things you can do as well as the more complicated emotional and philosophical stuff.

Understanding the anatomy (what goes where)

The brain consists of a large blob called the cerebrum, sitting on top of a stalk that joins to the spinal cord, with a bump hanging off the back called the cerebellum, as shown in Figure 4-1.

An adult brain weighs around 1.5 kilograms and has the consistency of tofu. It's made up of around 86 billion nerve cells, called neurons, arranged into two halves, called hemispheres, which are each divided further into four lobes: frontal, parietal, temporal and occipital.

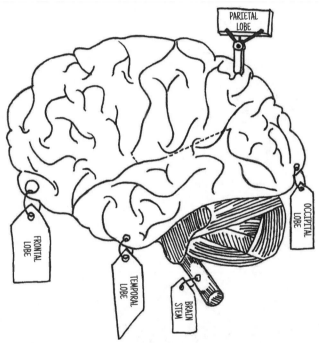

Figure 4-1:
The human brain.

Illustration by Sam Atkins

Neurons are the main components inside the brain. They're a bit like insulated wires carrying electrical signals around the brain to communicate between its different regions. Nerves (see Figure 4-2) pass these signals between each other at gaps called synapses (Figure 4-3). Here, the signal from one cell causes the release of chemicals across the synapse, which then attach to receptors on the next neuron, triggering a further electrical signal in the next cell, and so on; Figure 4-4 illustrates this process. Of these chemicals, called neurotransmitters, dopamine, glutamate and acetylcholine have the most relevance to dementia.

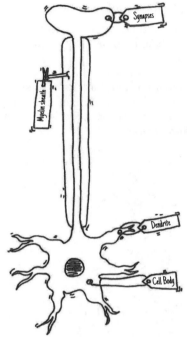

Figure 4-2:
A nerve cell.

Illustration by Sam Atkins

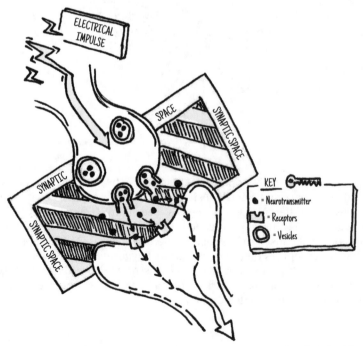

Figure 4-3:
A synapse.

Illustration by Sam Atkins

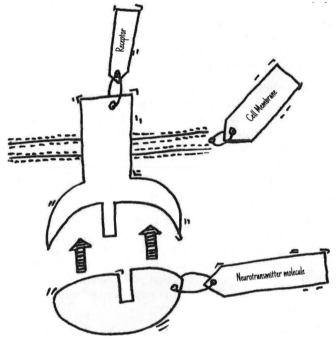

Figure 4-4:
A transmitter 'plugging' into a receptor.

Illustration by Sam Atkins

Fathoming functions (which bit does what)

In order to get a handle on what goes wrong in the brain in dementia, a basic knowledge of which bits of the brain are responsible for doing what is helpful. Here's a quick rundown:

- **Cerebral hemispheres:** The two cerebral hemispheres make up the majority of the structure of the brain. They're separated by a deep groove called the longitudinal fissure. The surface of the hemispheres, called the cortex, looks grey from the outside, hence the colloquial term for the brain: grey matter.

- **Frontal lobe:** Perhaps not surprisingly, given its name, this lobe is situated at the front of each hemisphere. This area is far more developed in humans than it is in other species of mammal, and it's where the higher intellectual functions are carried out, such as planning and mental reasoning. This part of the brain has allowed humans to evolve to the point of not only controlling their environment on earth but also sending rockets to the moon and beyond. The frontal lobe is also involved in speech and movement, and is the main centre for emotions.

✔ **Parietal lobe:** This area is involved in movement and, most importantly, houses the primary sensory cortex, which allows you to analyse and make sense of all the information that comes in from your sense organs. The parietal lobe is also the part of the brain that lets you know which way up you are in relation to the floor.

✔ **Temporal lobe:** This area of the brain is often affected in dementia. Given that it contains the hippocampus, which is involved in memory, it's not hard to see how memory problems are a significant feature of dementia. The temporal lobe also contains the primary auditory cortex, which deals with sound and hearing, and Wernicke's area, which allows you to understand speech and language.

✔ **Occipital lobe:** This part of the brain is involved in vision, allowing you to see shapes and colours.

✔ **Brain stem:** This is the most primitive part of the human brain and is found in one form or other in the brains of other, far less evolved creatures throughout the animal kingdom. It sits underneath the cerebral hemispheres and communicates directly with the spinal cord below it. It controls all the basic functions that you need to carry out unconsciously in order to stay alive, like breathing and a regular heartbeat. If this area of the brain is damaged, game over.

✔ **Cerebellum:** The cerebellum may look like a piece of cauliflower glued onto the back of the brain, but don't let looks deceive you. It's vital for balance, posture and co-ordination; when the cerebellum is prevented from doing its work properly, most commonly after a boozy night out, these functions just don't work.

✔ **Cerebrospinal fluid (CSF):** CSF circulates around the outside of the spinal cord and around and through the brain. It's the liquid that doctors are trying to get hold of when they do a lumbar puncture. CSF has two main jobs: removing the waste products made during metabolism by brain cells, and acting as a cushion, especially just under the skull, to protect the brain from damage during trauma (for example, after head injuries and car accidents).

✔ **Ventricles:** These are spaces within brain tissue through which CSF circulates. They're situated symmetrically in both hemispheres and enlarge in certain types of dementia as the brain cells around them shrink or die off.

✔ **Cortex:** The cortex isn't an area of the brain but rather the name for the outer level of cells that cover the brain. Depending on what lobe the cortex is in, it's involved in different functions, such as memory, thought, language and consciousness – all the things, in fact, that make you human.

Understanding how memory works

Here, I'm once again trying to simplify a subject that could fill a library and that's actually still somewhat mysterious despite the research techniques available to 21st-century science. That said, understanding a few of the basics helps you to make sense of what goes wrong in dementia.

Memory is obviously vital to normal functioning, hence the disability that results when it starts to fail. Without memory, you can't learn from or make links to the past, and so can't plan for the future. You can also get lost, not only geographically but also emotionally, while carrying out tasks and even in the middle of conversations. Lack of memory prevents you from being able to follow instructions and even to recognise those you love.

Humans have two main types of memory: short term and long term.

Short-term memory

Sometimes called working memory, the short-term memory allows you to remember things like telephone numbers or drinks orders at the bar. It has limited storage capacity, however, and empties quickly so that new items can be remembered.

People are thought to be able to retain lists of up to nine items for around 30 seconds in short-term memory before they're lost (unless those people repeat the items over and over again to try to hold on to them for longer). To retain memories for longer, they have to be transferred into the long-term memory, where storage is seemingly limitless and the memories can stay for the rest of your life.

Long-term memory

In the long-term memory, people lay down their memories for keeps: the address of your first home, the name of your primary school teacher, the FA Cup final score in 1974 (Liverpool 3, Newcastle United 0, in case you're interested), the recipe for Granny's lemon cake, Pythagoras's theorem and so on. Memories aren't stored in one particular part of the brain but involve the interaction and co-operation of a few different regions.

Long-term memory can be subdivided further into two main types:

- ✔ **Declarative memory:** This includes sights, sounds and smells from the past, phone numbers, general knowledge, meanings of words and memories of events that have happened to you.

- ✔ **Procedural memory:** This is the memory needed for performing tasks such as riding a bike, tying shoelaces and driving a car.

Memory processing

For memory to work, each of the following three stages has to happen:

1. **Encoding** (your ability to take in information)
2. **Storage**
3. **Retrieval**

A failure of all or any of these individual processes can cause memory impairment. Thus, for example, encoding and storage may be fine, but with no capacity for retrieval you won't recall what you've stored. Likewise, encoded information won't be retrieved if it wasn't stored. And so on.

Realising what goes wrong in dementia

Dementia interferes with the functioning of brain cells, which stops them communicating between each other and therefore carrying out their normal processes. The process of dementia inflicts two major types of damage on nerve cells, which then produce symptoms. First, the cells can be killed off or rendered largely inactive because they receive insufficient oxygen in the bloodstream, as in vascular dementia. Second, the internal workings of the cells themselves are messed up by protein deposits forming within them – that is, plaques and tangles in Alzheimer's disease, and Lewy bodies in Lewy body dementia.

Obviously, this is a simplistic view of things; it does, however, give you an idea of what can go wrong in an individual cell – although most often in large groups of cells – to impair how the whole brain works. This loss of function coupled with a reduction in levels of some of the neurotransmitters that let cells 'talk' to each other can thus cause large parts of a person's central nervous system to fail.

Not only is the type of damage important in generating symptoms in the different dementias, but where this damage occurs in the brain is also crucial in bringing about the changes observed in people with dementia. Each type of dementia has singular features, as well as more generalisable symptoms:

- ✔ **Fronto-temporal dementia:** The changes are mainly in the two fronto-temporal lobes, which are involved in both higher intellectual functions and memory processes. This damage then leads to the typical symptoms of dementia – from difficulty with planning and motivation to changes in personality and behaviour.

- ✔ **Alzheimer's disease:** The main area affected is the hippocampus, which is involved in converting short-term into long-term memories, hence the initial classic symptom whereby the person has difficulty remembering what's just happened. Memories already stored long term can, however, sometimes still be recalled.

> ✔ **Lewy body disease:** The damage is largely inflicted throughout the cortex, where Lewy bodies can be found in all the different lobes. Lewy bodies also crop up in the brain stem. Because the cortex is involved in both motor and sensory functions, people with Lewy body disease can develop hallucinations and difficulties with movement, leading to its particular cluster of symptoms.
>
> ✔ **Vascular dementia:** The areas that can be damaged are even more widespread still, given that blockages to blood supply or reductions in its flow can happen pretty much anywhere. Thus if the hippocampus is damaged, memory is affected; if the frontal lobes are involved, issues with planning and personality develop; and if strokes are the cause, movement can be impaired, resulting in paralysis.

The brain being the complicated organ that it is, the symptoms of the different types of dementia aren't quite as well demarcated as this, and many different areas can be involved in certain processes, especially memory. Damage to connecting cells between lobes can thus also result in difficulties.

Taking age into account

If I had a pound for every patient who's said to me 'old age doesn't come alone', I'd have more money than Simon Cowell and would currently be sitting on a sun-drenched beach on an island in the Indian Ocean. Sadly, those words of wisdom are always given to me for free. I do hear them a lot, however, and that's because they're true. As people age, they start to wear out: your eyesight deteriorates behind cloudy cataracts; your joints become arthritic and creak and groan when you move, stand, sit or do pretty much anything else; your hearing and hair (if you're a man) desert you; and you lose energy, sex drive and often mental sharpness. *But*, contrary to popular belief, not everyone develops dementia.

On the flip side, while it does become a more common occurrence with advancing years, dementia isn't limited to the ageing generation; some younger people can fall victim to it too. Although the Alzheimer's Society (www.alzheimers.org.uk) estimates that 1 in 14 people over the age of 65 will develop dementia, its statistics also show that 17,000 of the 800,000 people with dementia in the UK are under this age. And given that the Alzheimer's Society also reckons that only 44 per cent of people with dementia in England, Wales and Northern Ireland have actually been diagnosed, this number is likely to rise as pick-up rates improve.

The distribution of the different types of dementia is funnel shaped. At the top, the funnel is at its widest because for younger people the cause of dementia can be any one of the following: Alzheimer's disease, vascular dementia, Lewy body disease or fronto-temporal dementia. As a person's age at time of diagnosis goes up, the funnel narrows towards its point, because over the age of 75 most people diagnosed with dementia are diagnosed with Alzheimer's disease, with some cases of mixed dementia thrown in too.

Understanding the Role of Genes and Family History

Unfortunately, many medical conditions run in families and are thus passed on from one generation to the next simply by the act of reproduction rather than being picked up from elsewhere or developed because of bad habits. Common examples are colour-blindness and, more rarely, Huntington's disease.

Many more conditions don't develop automatically but are more likely to develop in someone given the right (or wrong in this case) conditions as a result of genetic predisposition. A mental health problem such as schizophrenia, which may only develop if someone experiences particularly difficult life events, is one such example.

Explaining what genes are and how they work

Each person has between 20,000 and 25,000 genes in her body. Genes are found within each of your cells; you can think of them as the blueprint for how people are put together. Thus you have genes that dictate your hair colour, the shape of your nose, ears and feet, how tall you become, whether you have a hairy chest and, of course, whether you're male or female. These genes are bundled up on your chromosomes. Everyone has 23 pairs of chromosomes, making 46 in total; half come from your mother, and half from your father.

Your genes, and therefore your chromosomes, are made of a chemical called deoxyribonucleic acid, or DNA for short. DNA is itself made up of four different types of protein molecule:

- ✔ Adenine (A)
- ✔ Cytosine (C)
- ✔ Guanine (G)
- ✔ Thymine (T)

DNA comes as long strands of these proteins that provide the code for hair colour and so on, depending upon the order they occur in. So, for example, a gene (which in reality would be much, much longer) with the order AGTACCCTTACGACT would code for one characteristic, while

CCCGTTATATGCTA would code for another. The process is obviously much more complicated than that, but hopefully this example gives you the idea. Figure 4-5 illustrates how DNA forms genes and then chromosomes.

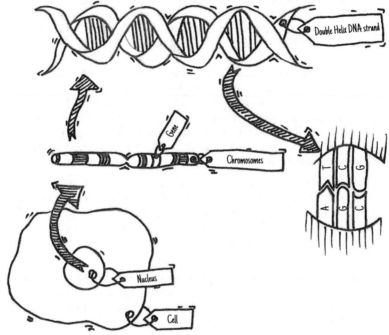

Figure 4-5: How DNA forms genes and then chromosomes.

Illustration by Sam Atkins

In an ideal world, your DNA would be perfect and your genes and chromosomes would give you only healthy characteristics, movie-star good looks and the gift of eternal life. However, disease is rife, most people don't look in the mirror and see Angelina Jolie or Brad Pitt looking back, and everyone dies one day, some people sooner than others. Actually, during the process of evolution, these genetic abnormalities have worked to the advantage of the species, making some people stronger, brighter or better looking than others, and thus enabling the human race to advance. Unfortunately, the other side of that coin is that genes that disadvantage people can also be passed on to the next generation and cause disease.

The fact that half your genes come from one parent and half from the other does provide the opportunity for 'bad' genes to die out. However, some people still suffer from conditions that run in the family.

Identifying whether dementia runs in families

I'm frequently asked by relatives of people with dementia whether I think they'll develop it too. Unfortunately, no easy, straightforward answer exists, and even the experts aren't clear about the genetics of each type of dementia. The case is different for each sort of dementia:

- **Alzheimer's disease:** The situation depends on whether someone has early- or late-onset Alzheimer's. A very rare type of early-onset Alzheimer's disease exists that definitely runs in families, with some members developing symptoms as young as 30. This type is caused by a mutation in the gene that makes amyloid protein, which is responsible for the plaques and tangles that form in sufferers' brain cells. People in these families are advised to see their doctor to arrange genetic testing.

   In the case of late-onset dementia, you may possibly but by no means definitely develop Alzheimer's disease if you have a relative with the condition. The gene responsible is apolipoprotein E (APOE for short), which is found on chromosome number 19. This gene has four variants, and the likelihood of the disease being passed on depends on which of these variants a person has.

- **Vascular dementia:** No proven genetic risk exists for most cases of vascular dementia, although its associated risk factors, such as heart disease and diabetes, can run in families. The only exception to this is CADASIL, which is a rare genetic form of the condition.

- **Fronto-temporal dementia:** In contrast to vascular dementia, there is a risk of fronto-temporal dementia running in families. Researchers have identified genes for two different abnormal proteins that could be responsible for this. It is reckoned that around 40 per cent of people with fronto-temporal dementia have a family history.

   If you have a close relative with fronto-temporal dementia, seek genetic counselling via your GP.

- **Lewy body dementia:** No clear answer can be given to the question of whether a genetic component exists in the development of this form of dementia. Some overlap in genetic mutations with those who have Alzheimer's disease and Parkinson's disease is thought to be evident, but no one can yet say for certain.

Interestingly, dementia doesn't discriminate. It affects people from all ethnic backgrounds. In the UK the numbers of people from some particular ethnic groups do appear low, but that's the result of other factors, including

- Access to services

- Poor experiences when seeking help from GPs

✔ Cultural understanding of the condition

✔ Stigma attached to being given the diagnosis

Hopefully, this situation will change so that people can receive the treatment and care they need regardless of their ethnic background.

Taking a Long, Hard Look at the Risk Factors

Everyone loves a conspiracy theory. If you believed all the newspaper headlines about the risks various pollutants, drugs, cosmetics and foodstuffs pose to your health and very survival, you'd never venture outside the front door. But whether truth exists in any of it – and particularly whether dementia can be triggered by factors in your everyday environment – remains an open question.

I've scoured the Internet and the research journals to make sure I'm not missing anything, but I think I can safely say that although you should always be careful about what you swallow and breathe in, no clear evidence suggests that environmental factors are involved in developing dementia. Air pollution may apparently predispose older people to cognitive decline, but no link has yet been made to a progression to dementia.

Lifestyle

Here, at last, I may have come across some factors with actual proven risk and that you can do something about from a prevention point of view. No one lives a completely healthy lifestyle all the time. I may run marathons and take part in 100-mile bike rides, but I still enjoy a pasty and a pint.

The infamous case of aluminium

In 1965 some very creative, not to mention cruel, scientists carried out an experiment whereby they injected rabbits' brains with aluminium. At post-mortem, the animal-friendly scientists found that the rabbits had developed the textbook neurofibrillary protein tangles that are found in the brains of people with Alzheimer's disease. And so began the story linking the third-most common chemical element on the planet with the most common form of dementia.

Since then all sorts of scares have suggested that even using aluminium saucepans or deodorants containing the stuff will lead to dementia. After years of research, this link hasn't been proved, and currently aluminium is viewed as safe. Just don't inject it directly into your brain!

However, the factors listed below won't surprise anyone. Doctors and nurses bang on about these issues every time someone has an appointment. The government commissions adverts warning against them, and the walls of every health centre and clinic in the country are decorated with posters that promote a healthy lifestyle that includes

- ✔ Not taking drugs (other than caffeine, and that in moderation)
- ✔ Drinking less alcohol
- ✔ Not smoking
- ✔ Eating more fruit and fibre
- ✔ Eating fewer burgers
- ✔ Doing more exercise

Drugs and alcohol

Flippancy aside, illicit drugs are bad – full stop. I've yet to meet a patient who's had a serious drug habit and emerged unscathed. Evidence supporting a link between street drugs and full-on dementia is flimsy at best; however, cannabis, heroin, ecstasy, amphetamines and cocaine are known to cause cognitive impairment.

Alcohol can cause its own form of dementia, Korsakoff's syndrome. Try to stick to current recommended daily intakes: three to four units per day for a man and two to three for a woman. If you're gulping down more than that a day, you need to have a chat with your GP about getting help to reduce your intake. Not only does alcohol increase your risk of developing dementia, but it also rots pretty much every organ in the body.

Smoking

If I could sum up my advice on smoking in one word, it would be *don't*. Smoking is the biggest risk factor for every form of premature death known to medical science, from cancer of every organ in your body (no exaggeration) to heart attack and stroke. The habit also doubles your risk of dementia, especially Alzheimer's disease and vascular dementia, by damaging brain cells and blood vessels.

Thankfully, lots of things are available to help you stop, such as nicotine-replacement therapies, pills, patches, electronic cigarettes, hypnosis, pills – all obtainable from your GP, practice nurse or a pharmacist. Your GP practice can even point you in the direction of a support group if you think you'll struggle alone.

If you want to avoid dementia and don't have a strong family history of the disease, quitting cigarettes will do you far more good than chucking out your aluminium saucepans.

Diet

People who are obese are four times more likely to develop dementia than those who aren't overweight. People who eat foods that are high in fat are in general more at risk of damaging their blood vessels and thus reducing the blood supply to the brain, making them more at risk of dementia.

A diet low in fat and high in fibre is best. Eating five portions of fruit and vegetables per day is strongly recommended. Doing so reduces the risk of furring up your arteries, and these foods are also rich in antioxidants, which protect brain cells from damage.

If you're a man, aim to eat less than 30 grams of saturated fat each day; if you're a woman, aim for less than 20. Laying off fatty meats, pies, full-fat dairy products like cheese and butter, as well as chocolate, crisps and biscuits certainly helps. Foods laden with fibre include wholegrain bread, brown rice, beans, peas, lentils, nuts and cereals containing bran. To maintain a healthy diet, experts suggest an intake of 18 grams of fibre per day.

Exercise

Not only does taking regular exercise fend off heart disease, but it can also protect against Alzheimer's disease and vascular dementia. Fortunately, this doesn't mean that you have to rush out and join a gym, deck yourself out in Lycra or sign up to run the London Marathon. Obviously, you can if you like, but five half-hour sessions of brisk walking every week will do you just as much good.

Get off the bus a couple of stops early, take the stairs rather than the lift or walk the dog every day.

Swimming, cycling, aerobics and many other forms of exercise can help, but you really don't need to do more than add in a bit more sweat to your normal daily routine.

Putting risk in perspective

We don't live in a risk-free world. You only have to watch the news to see how unlucky people can be when they're partaking in seemingly low-risk pursuits. A Brazilian fan died from a heart attack just watching a penalty shoot-out during the 2014 World Cup, for example. Conversely, even if you're placed in a high-risk category in terms of developing dementia, you may still get lucky and avoid it, particularly if you look after yourself and remain in good health.

You're probably at greater risk of dying in an accident than you are of succumbing to dementia. So look both ways when you cross the road, quit smoking and skydiving and always wear a seat belt – you'll probably be fine.

Mental stimulation

So-called brain-training exercises are big business. You can buy brain-training apps for your phone or tablet, and programs for every kind of games console. If you keep your brain active doing these tests, so the spiel goes, your general cognitive function will improve too.

Sadly, research doesn't support this claim. In fact, according to various dementia charities, learning new skills, trying out different hobbies and doing crosswords, Sudoku and other puzzles do far more good. Socialising with others can also protect your brain from cognitive decline – so join a poker club, take up salsa or set up a book group.

Chapter 5

Understanding the Stages of Dementia

In This Chapter

▶ Working through the three stages of dementia

▶ Exploring the progression of different types of dementia

Dementia, in all its manifestations, is a progressive disease. And although this decline is most often seen as a continuous process rather than happening in phases, dividing up its course into early, middle and late stages to get a better idea of how symptoms change over the course of the disease is useful.

Unsurprisingly, the edges of these stages are blurred, and each individual experiences dementia differently, depending on his pre-illness personality, the other medical conditions he may have and whether he receives good support. However, the stages I describe are still a good general guide to what to expect in the months and years after diagnosis.

I start by looking at dementia in general, using Alzheimer's disease as my main example, and end by looking at any specific peculiarities seen in vascular dementia, fronto-temporal dementia and Lewy body disease.

Looking at the Early Stage

This stage has particularly blurred edges, because it contains some of the very first symptoms someone may exhibit as he develops dementia. These may be new symptoms appearing out of the blue or a progression from longer-standing mild cognitive impairment. Either way, symptoms are likely to develop in a different order and at different speeds in different people. Nonetheless, the sections below describe the behaviours and symptoms to look out for.

Everyone is different, and dementia can express itself differently in all of us.

Knowing what to expect at the start

Life for doctors, patients and their families would be so much easier if diseases always followed their textbook descriptions to the letter. That way, diagnosing every medical condition would be a piece of cake, treatment could be started quickly and patients would be better off. But life's just not like that, in sickness or in health. And early dementia is no different.

People can exhibit dramatically different early symptoms. Some people show symptoms that initially baffle their doctors, and are medical mysteries for some time before the diagnostic penny drops (often because their symptoms could easily be due to a host of other conditions). Likewise, others pitch up at their GP's surgery and may as well have the diagnosis tattooed on their foreheads, it's so obvious to pick up.

But however it rears its head, early dementia has two main effects on someone: change and loss. Identifiable changes in memory, mood, personality and ability to manage day-to-day living will be evident. Not only does a person with early-stage dementia physically lose objects and bits of his memory, but you also notice that you're losing something of your relationship with him, as well as him losing aspects of what made him the person he is.

Expecting the unexpected is wise, because you can never be 100 per cent sure how dementia will announce itself.

Recognising the first signs of dementia

Most sufferers demonstrate most, but not necessarily all, of the following symptoms:

- ✔ **Memory loss:** This is the reason why most people take themselves, or are taken, to see the GP. Forgetting names, faces, dates, appointments, directions to familiar places and details of recent events is generally the problem.

- ✔ **Problems in conversation:** People regularly notice that their relative, friend or spouse has begun to have trouble following the thread of conversations when chatting to him and/or that he keeps saying the same things over and over again, as if for the first time, or repeating the same questions.

- ✔ **Difficulty managing change:** Any deviation from normal routine can become a struggle to deal with, as can adopting new ideas. This change is most noticeable in people who've always been up for a challenge or adaptable in relation to trying new ways of doing things. Likewise, stick-in-the-muds can become even more stuck and set in their ways. Another early sign may be dithering longer over making decisions such as where to go on holiday and choosing between two items to buy when out shopping, what to have from the menu in a restaurant and which clothes to wear to work or out for the evening.

✔ **Losing things:** This behaviour can become the rule rather than the exception in early dementia, and can include regularly misplacing items like keys, reading glasses and television remote controls.

✔ **Poor judgement:** Simple monetary transactions can become confusing, and people with early dementia are also more likely to fall for a bargain or sign up for an insurance policy or mobile phone contract they don't need.

✔ **Alteration of mood:** Low mood, anxiety, uncertainty, mood swings, irritability and a withdrawal from usual social activities can all be early symptoms of dementia.

Considering the Middle Stage

Apologies for sounding a little repetitive about the unpredictability of dementia, but the time between the start of the early stage of dementia and its progression into the middle stage can vary dramatically. It would obviously be a lot tidier if each stage lasted a set number of years, to allow sufferers and their carers to plan ahead with some degree of accuracy. But dementia isn't that accommodating, and while many people may dawdle along in the early stage for many years, others can sprint through it and show a deterioration in their symptoms quite quickly.

Acknowledging that dementia has set in

In the middle stage, the symptoms that have sporadically appeared and perhaps fluctuated in the first stage become more permanent and their arrival also gathers pace. As a result, people in this stage regularly have memory problems, develop difficulties with day-to-day functions like cooking, shopping and dressing, and demonstrate much more obvious changes in their mood and behaviour.

It becomes increasingly obvious that these changes can't simply be put down to senior moments or the perceived inevitability of a progression towards eccentricity and increased grumpiness as old age sets in. At this stage, it's clear that something's wrong, and medical advice about what's going on and what can be done about it is now essential.

Realising how symptoms evolve

The symptoms demonstrated in the first stage now become more extreme, and the following may be more likely:

- **Memory loss:** This symptom becomes more severe and sufferers regularly forget names of family members and friends, miss appointments and often put themselves and others at risk by, for example, leaving pans cooking on the stove, eating food that's well out of date or going out and leaving the front door open.

- **Problems in conversation:** Repetition can become the norm in conversation, or people in the middle stage of dementia may not bother to join in, because they simply can't follow what's been said. They may also have trouble finding the right words for things, so describe them instead; thus a watch, for example, becomes 'the time-telling thing on my arm'. People at this stage are also prone to confabulation – filling in memory gaps with false details that they believe to be true. If asked what they did at the weekend, for example, they provide a description of events that bears no resemblance to the truth, but is nonetheless a plausible reply.

- **Losing things:** In the middle stage of dementia, the most common things to become lost may well be the dementia sufferers themselves. Wandering is common and leads to people being unable to find their way to their proposed destination or their way home. Losing track of whether it's day or night isn't unusual, and heading outside in pyjamas may be a regular occurrence.

- **Alteration of mood:** Depression, anger and irritability can be more prominent, as can elated and disinhibited behaviour, leading to the person making inappropriate and even sexual suggestions to strangers. Anxiety is also seen in this stage, most often manifested in following loved ones around and constantly seeking reassurance from them.

- **Suspicious minds:** Paranoia and suspicion are frequent features of this stage of dementia, often leading to aggression towards others who are believed to have stolen things from the sufferer or to be out to get him.

- **Self-care:** Personal hygiene often suffers in this stage of dementia, and people need to be prompted to change dirty clothes, wash and shower, and brush their teeth. They may also begin to develop incontinence, which compounds the problem of staying clean and tidy.

Identifying the Late Stage

By now, the effects of dementia are severe. Sufferers in this stage may well be totally dependent on others for their daily care, and may already be in a nursing or care home. Symptoms again vary between people, but they're heading towards the end of their days.

Knowing it's the final chapter

At this point, the person with dementia succumbs to the full force of the effects of the disease, completely dispelling the myth that dementia is simply a memory problem. In this final stage, while a severe loss of memory is definitely evident, an erosion of much of the capacity to exist in any meaningful way as an independent individual occurs and, existentially, a loss of self results.

Unfortunately, intellectual effects aren't the only signs of this stage of dementia: it also plays havoc with the sufferer's physical capabilities too. Not only are sufferers often incapable of carrying out the most basic activities of daily life, but they also become physically frail, at high risk of falls and extremely susceptible to serious infections.

Again, exceptions to this pattern of deterioration always exist, but for most people in the late stage of dementia any faculties that haven't already been lost or shut down pretty quickly begin to now. This change manifests itself in a number of ways:

- ✔ Physical frailty may lead to confinement to, initially, a wheelchair and, ultimately, to bed.

- ✔ Feeding can be a problem, compounded by swallowing difficulties, and severe weight loss may result.

- ✔ Memory is very limited, and while occasional moments of clear reminiscence may occur, it's more common for people in this stage to have little recollection of day-to-day events, names of objects and, most upsetting for families, names of their nearest and dearest.

- ✔ Speech can be lost, so that people with severe dementia may only utter individual words and sounds, often repetitively. They also lose the ability to understand the words of others, and meaningful conversation thus becomes nigh-on impossible.

- ✔ Agitation and irritability can be common, with refusal to co-operate with carers being a frequent issue. Shouting, lashing out with hands and fists, pulling hair and biting are possible responses to well-intentioned offers of help. It's not unusual for family members and spouses to find this extreme rejection of their best efforts to reach out to their loved one very upsetting and particularly difficult to deal with emotionally.

Moving towards the end of life

The daughter of one of my patients once said to me, as we sat at her mother's bedside, that she felt she'd lost her mother to dementia a long time ago, and was just waiting for her body to catch up so that she could start grieving properly. That's a common feeling among relatives and friends of a person in the final stage of dementia and, thankfully, the end of life isn't far away.

And I say thankfully not only from my own clinical experience of dealing with my patients and their families, but from personal experience too. My uncle and grandmother experienced different forms of dementia, and when they reached the stage where it had robbed them of their minds, their physical strength and their identities, it was a relief when they finally passed away.

In the late stage of dementia, sufferers are more susceptible to certain health problems than are people of the same age who don't have dementia. Death may result from a number of causes, such as

✔ Falls leading to fractures, plus poor healing and/or complications following surgery to repair such fractures. Stress experienced as a result of the trauma and the experience of being in hospital may also prove fatal.

✔ Infections such as pneumonia, urinary-tract infections or skin infections resulting from bed sores.

✔ Progressive deterioration in general health as a result of poor nutrition and weakness.

While death is likely to be hastened by any of the causes listed, it's also extremely common for people with dementia simply to give up on life and pass away peacefully as a result of increasing frailty. Death need not be traumatic; in Chapter 20 I look in more detail at end-of-life planning and palliative care for someone with dementia, because it's as important for someone to have a 'good death' as it is for him to enjoy a good life.

Exploring Variations in Other Types of Dementia

So far in this chapter I've used what happens to people with Alzheimer's disease as the template for the changes that happen to people with dementia. Most people largely follow this pattern. However, given the differences in symptoms caused by the other types of dementia, a quick look at how these conditions can produce their own idiosyncratic changes in sufferers is worthwhile.

Vascular dementia

Given that the underlying cause of vascular dementia is often recurrent strokes or transient ischaemic attacks, each time sufferers experience another one, their condition further deteriorates. As a result, progression in this kind of dementia can be stepwise rather than smooth and gradual, with significant changes occurring in a person's symptoms after each new episode.

However, a stepwise progression isn't always the case, because vascular dementia can also be caused by the slow but progressive process of hardening of the arteries (atherosclerosis). And if that's the case, symptoms are also more likely to develop slowly and progressively, as they do in Alzheimer's disease.

A third, very positive, possibility also exists: if the person has no more strokes, his symptoms may not deteriorate significantly at all.

The other main difference in vascular dementia is that the areas of the brain affected by the strokes are those that produce symptoms, and other areas may thus remain unaffected. This can make the symptoms and disabilities caused by the condition less extensive than those of Alzheimer's, in which the effects are much more global.

In the later stages of vascular dementia, the symptoms are largely the same as in Alzheimer's. Research suggests, however, that because personality is often preserved to a greater degree in vascular dementia, people with the condition can be more aware of their predicament and consequently more prone to depression.

The other big difference in vascular dementia is cause of death, which, because of the person's underlying problems with the circulatory system, is often a heart attack or stroke.

Fronto-temporal dementia

The biggest difference between fronto-temporal and other types of dementia is that it can happen a lot earlier in life, often in middle age rather than old age. Obvious and specific features of this condition are often related to interpersonal skills:

- ✔ Apathy
- ✔ Sexual and social disinhibition
- ✔ Obsessions and rituals

People may also, seemingly out of the blue, switch jobs or partners and change dietary or musical preferences.

The other big difference is that memory can often still be pretty good in the early stages. As the condition progresses, however, development of symptoms gathers momentum and memory does become an issue.

In the later stages, people with fronto-temporal dementia may have the following issues:

- Wandering
- Apathy and sometimes mutism
- Incontinence
- Swallowing difficulties

The situation otherwise is similar to that experienced by people with Alzheimer's disease. Life expectancy is six to eight years after symptoms first develop.

Lewy body disease

The unique feature of Lewy body disease in its early stage is the way in which someone's intellectual abilities and levels of confusion can fluctuate, not only from day to day, but also within the course of the same 24-hour period. And as with fronto-temporal dementia, memory problems aren't such a major issue as they are in early Alzheimer's disease.

As the disease progresses into its middle to late stages, its stand-out symptoms are

- Visual hallucinations
- Spontaneous features of Parkinson's disease, affecting mobility
- Repeated falls, fainting and occasionally episodes of passing out
- Acting out dreams – rapid eye movement (REM) sleep behaviour disorder
- Swallowing problems

These symptoms mean that by the time the disease is in its later stages sufferers need round-the-clock care and are so restricted physically that they're likely to be bed-bound. Death is often caused by a severe chest infection (pneumonia) triggered by the swallowing difficulties that channel food and drink into the lungs rather than directly into the stomach.

The high risk of falls can also mean that people are extremely susceptible to fractures and head injuries. As a result, life expectancy is on average five to seven years following diagnosis.

Life expectancy after diagnosis of dementia

The big question on everyone's lips when they're diagnosed with a life-limiting illness is, of course, 'How long have I got, Doc?' And it's a question I hate having to answer, not simply because my estimate may be a lot shorter than the timescale they're hoping for, but also because my estimate is invariably wrong. Humans rarely play by the rules suggested by the textbooks, because so many factors can play a part in determining each individual's outcome.

As biologist Richard Dawkins says, we humans are 'survival machines' for our genes; to enable them to be successfully passed on from generation to generation, we've evolved some pretty good mechanisms to ensure our survival. These mechanisms have done our species proud since we first evolved in the sunshine of East Africa 200,000 years ago.

So it's never as simple as saying, 'If you have diagnosis A, you'll therefore live X number of months,' because so many other factors come into play, including

- The stage the condition has reached before it's picked up

- Age at diagnosis

- Other health conditions

- Tolerance of treatment provided for the condition

- Psychological impact, and the patient's general state of mind

- The strength of the patient's immune system

- Social circumstances and levels of deprivation

I had a patient with cancer who was told her condition was so severe that she literally had just a few weeks to live. She was given one last throw of the dice in the form of a final dose of chemotherapy, and was miraculously cured. In contrast, another patient given a much less severe diagnosis took to his bed, shut himself off from friends and family and died in his sleep not long after.

Dementia is no different, and people's responses to it vary. But having a rough idea of what to expect can be helpful in planning for the future, hence the frequency of the 'How long have I got?' question. In broad terms, therefore, the outlook is generally not good. A study published in the *British Medical Journal* in 2008 found that the average survival time after diagnosis was 4.6 years for women and 4.1 years for men. But that's a very cautious average, and the various dementia charities suggest that life expectancy ranges from 3.5 years from diagnosis at its shortest to 20 years at its longest, with people who are older when diagnosed being at the lower end of the scale.

Bearing in mind that the period from development to diagnosis spans an average 2.8 years, an actual figure is, unfortunately, always hard to predict.

Part II

Helping Someone Manage the Illness

The top five ways to deal with dementia

- ✔ **See the doctor.** Your GP is the best person to get the ball rolling about whether your symptoms are dementia related and, if so, to which type of dementia.

- ✔ **Stay in touch with your local surgery.** The involvement of your family doctor doesn't stop at a diagnosis. GPs can advise on medication to help slow the progress of the condition and can enlist the help of nurses and social services in your care, as and when needed.

- ✔ **Try medication.** Although, sadly, no cure for dementia exists, a handful of drugs is available from your GP or dementia specialist that may alleviate your symptoms.

- ✔ **Explore some complementary therapies.** A range of these therapies is on offer, from aromatherapy to music and reminiscence therapies, which not only help to calm someone when she's distressed but also help you to connect with her and improve her quality of life.

- ✔ **Get in touch with the local authority.** Get a range of support services from meals on wheels to home care staff who help make life easier for the person with dementia as her condition progresses.

Get more information about how dementia is diagnosed and the tests that are involved at www.dummies.com/extras/dementia.

In this part . . .

✔ Find out what to expect following a trip to the doctor's to discuss the possibility of dementia and the kinds of tests that might be involved in determining a diagnosis.

✔ Discover the strengths and limitations of the medicines that doctors can prescribe to help slow down the progress of dementia.

✔ Review the wealth of alternative therapies claimed to help dementia and look at the evidence for whether they're worth trying or not.

✔ Get hints and tips for dealing with some of the more tricky symptoms that can occur in the later stages of dementia.

Chapter 6

Getting a Diagnosis

· ·

In This Chapter

▶ Working through the stages to gain a diagnosis

▶ Understanding what happens post diagnosis

▶ Planning ongoing care

· ·

*V*ery often, not knowing what's wrong with you, or someone you care for, is worse than actually knowing. That may sound a bit odd because, for example, not knowing you have cancer is surely a better state to be in than being told you have the diagnosis. Without the information you're just a person with a few symptoms, but once you have a diagnosis you're a cancer patient, with operations, chemotherapy or radiotherapy ahead of you and a rough answer to the inevitable question: how long have I got left?

But as many of my patients who themselves have been given all manner of difficult diagnoses have testified, once a set of symptoms has a name, once you've been told that you have this or that disease, you and your family know what you're up against. In fact, people often say that the worry of not knowing is far worse than the worry associated with knowing what's wrong.

With a label to your illness comes a treatment plan, the knowledge that medical teams are going to do their best to look after you, and if not make you better then at least take away the worst of your symptoms. Without a label, you often imagine even worse diagnoses than the one you're about to be given. Anxiety about the condition also makes the likely outlook seem worse, as you envisage all sorts of catastrophic scenarios about symptoms and treatments.

And, of course, with many diseases the sooner you get a diagnosis, the more likely it is that you can be cured. Sadly, with all types of dementia, there's no cure, no matter how soon the condition is picked up. But early diagnosis does mean that some medicines may help keep symptoms at bay for longer, and it certainly gives more time to plan long-term care.

Taking the First Step towards a Diagnosis

In this chapter I look at the initial steps that you need to take in order to find out whether you're dealing with dementia or whether something else is responsible for the symptoms you or a loved one are experiencing. Because this book is intended for readers throughout the UK, it must be noted that the situation in different parts of the country may well vary from those I describe. However, as the government continues to place a high priority on services for people with dementia, the hope is that these services will become more uniform, with better training for professionals dealing with the condition and greater access to both diagnostic tests and follow-up treatment and care.

Wherever you live in the UK, the first port of call on your journey is an appointment at the GP's surgery.

Seeing the GP

People in the UK are in the very fortunate situation of having a government-funded national health service – the NHS – which is free at the point of need for everyone. Everyone, no matter how rich or poor, old or young, is entitled to free access to a family doctor who can advise about all aspects of physical and mental health.

GPs have full copies of all your medical records since birth and so are well placed to use this knowledge of your background medical history to make new diagnoses. Using the service to the best of your advantage is important, because seeing the wrong person, or combinations of doctors, can slow down the process and lead to confusion for both patient and doctor.

Picking the right doctor

All GPs have been through extensive training following their graduation from medical school. This training includes time spent working on those specialist hospital wards relevant to being a family doctor, such as

- Emergency medicine
- Elderly care
- Psychiatry
- Obstetrics and gynaecology
- Paediatrics

Trainee GPs also spend a further 18 months in GP surgeries under the tutelage of a GP trainer, to hone the very different and particular skills needed to work as a doctor in general practice. The trainee GP then has to pass some pretty tough examinations validated by the Royal College of General Practitioners before she can put her name on a metal plate outside a surgery and work as a fully fledged GP. So whoever you choose to see in your local surgery, you can be assured that she's fully qualified to give you the best advice available and that if she does not have the answers to all your queries, she will know the relevant professionals to pass you on to.

However, you need to consider a number of factors when picking, from among the group at your practice, the particular doctor you want to see about your potential case of dementia. In making your choice, consider the answers to these questions:

- ✔ **Does she know you?** If you have a regular doctor who's known you for years, treated every cough and pulled muscle, seen you through antenatal care or your vasectomy, and poked her latex-gloved fingers into places where strangers would never dare, then you should start with her. Her wealth of background knowledge about your health and normal personality makes her able to pick up changes in you that help her come to a diagnosis or, conversely, to reassure you that nothing she's seen in your appointment alarms her.

- ✔ **Does she have a special interest in dementia?** Although sadly not the norm, a few practices have a lead GP for dementia care. The doctor has done extra training in the symptoms and signs of the condition and its treatment, and is well placed to give the best information about it. She often has close links with a community dementia nurse with whom she can discuss any queries about your case. Because she works in the same practice as your usual GP, the lead GP for dementia care can discuss your case with your GP if she needs any background information.

- ✔ **Has she helped someone you know with the condition?** You may not have darkened a doctor's doorstep for years, other than perhaps for flu vaccines or holiday jabs. If that's the case, a recommendation from a relative, friend or neighbour about which doctor to see can be helpful. If this person has found a doctor who's knowledgeable about dementia or particularly sympathetic, booking to see her is worthwhile.

- ✔ **Which doctor do the receptionists suggest?** If you're brand new to an area and have no knowledge of the doctors at the local surgery, ask at reception. Doctors' receptionists aren't all dragons, as they're portrayed in the media, and will be very happy to help point you in the right direction. They'll always find somewhere quiet to speak to you if you want to talk in confidence without the rest of the waiting room listening in.

Ensuring continuity

When you've decided on the doctor you want to see, and are happy with her, stick with her. Continuity of care is crucial when you have a chronic condition such as dementia. The doctor who sees you has a working knowledge of the situation, a handle on the investigations performed so far and a plan in her head about how to progress. This plan is individualised to you. A different doctor, without all the facts at her fingertips or the luxury of having a thorough background knowledge of you, may have a different plan. Seeing different GPs at different times may make your management far more complicated and fragmented than it need be.

Even if you need to see a doctor for an unplanned appointment, always try to wait for your own to be available rather than seeing someone else (unless it's an emergency, of course). This advice also applies to situations that occur out of hours at the weekends or on bank holidays. Unless it's a medical emergency and therefore life-threatening or it may mean an immediate trip to hospital, try to wait to see your usual doctor.

With the best will in the world but working without a full set of your medical records, an emergency doctor is more likely to be over-cautious about your symptoms than someone who knows you. If you see a doctor who doesn't know you, you may be prescribed unnecessary pills, given tests you may not need or have already had or, worse still, you may end up taking a precautionary trip to hospital, to sit on a trolley in accident and emergency for the rest of the day.

Of course, if you're facing an emergency or are in a pickle you can't work your way out of, you must ring for help. But always be mindful that, as is the case with cooks and spoilt broth, too many doctors can mess things up and leave a bad taste in your mouth.

Considering what the doctor wants to know

My professors at medical school always maintained that 80 per cent of any diagnosis can be made from taking a good medical history alone. A thorough physical examination then almost clinches it, with blood tests and scans simply putting the icing on the diagnostic cake. So whereas doctors on TV may shout for x-rays the moment a patient walks through the hospital door, their real-life counterparts want to ask a few questions.

The current situation

A bit like journalists getting the full details for their scoop, doctors want to know many of the five Ws and an H that are crucial to a news story: who, what, where, why, when and how? You can help your doctor with her information gathering by writing things down and taking your notes to the appointment with you.

Specifically, the doctor wants to know:

- **Why have you booked an appointment today?** What's changed or become worse and made you want to see a doctor? Was the visit precipitated by a friend, neighbour or family member who's noticed a worrying change in you?

- **What are the symptoms?** This is your chance, and that of anyone you've chosen to take with you to the appointment, to have your say. Don't worry about trying to use clever medical terms to describe what's been happening; the doctor wants you to get it across to her in your own words and not sound as though you've eaten a medical dictionary for breakfast. Tell her whatever is worrying you, and don't forget that she wants to know about physical problems just as much as those affecting your memory and thought processes.

- **When did the symptoms start?** The doctor not only wants an idea of how long you've been struggling for but also whether the symptoms started suddenly or crept up on you gradually, and whether they've become slowly worse or changed in a stepwise pattern. It also helps to know whether anything else was going on in your life at the time your symptoms started, such as a bereavement or an accident involving a head injury. All this information is helpful in the diagnostic process.

- **Who first noticed the symptoms?** Very often you're the first to notice when your brain or body starts to play up. You may notice that you're more out of breath than usual when running for the bus, or spot a change in the way your bowels are working, or feel a new lump that's popped up somewhere embarrassing. But where dementia's concerned, often someone else at home or work notices that you're becoming forgetful, starting to frequently lose things or getting in a muddle when carrying out tasks you previously performed with your eyes closed.

- **How are the symptoms affecting you in day-to-day life?** Dementia isn't just about memory: it can also lead to changes in mood and the way you carry out ordinary, day-to-day tasks. So tell the doctor if you're having difficulty completing the cryptic crossword you previously whistled through without a hitch, or how preparing a meal has become tricky.

The doctor then homes in on your answers to find out more about each issue. So, for example, if you've mentioned a problem with baking cakes, she'll want to know which parts of the process have become most troublesome. Is it, for example, remembering the recipe, physically stirring the mixture or setting a timer on the cooker so that the cake doesn't burn?

Because these things can be difficult to remember well if you have a memory problem, it's often a good idea to write down a list of points you want to get across in answer to these sorts of questions, and take the list with you. You can also go with a friend or relative who has a good understanding of the situation.

Background history

Even with the medical notes on the computer screen in front of her, your doctor's likely to want to ask some questions that give your current symptoms some background context and detail. Getting things straight from the horse's mouth is a good idea anyway, because it enables the doctor to fill in gaps in your record.

The doctor particularly wants to know about

- **Family history of similar conditions:** These questions focus on how distantly related the affected people were and how often the problem has cropped up.

- **Social history:** These questions address whether you smoke, how much alcohol you drink and what your hobbies are (and if those hobbies are affected).

- **Dietary history:** These questions deal with your appetite and whether you have dietary restrictions or particular habits such as drinking gallons of coffee every day or eating only hamburgers while skipping all your five-a-day fruit and vegetables.

- **Educational and occupational history:** These questions investigate how you did at school, how long you remained in education and what sort of job you have or had. (Insights into how your symptoms affect your work are particularly useful.)

Thinking about the examinations and tests the doctor performs

Once the doctor has all the information she needs about your symptoms and history, she'll move on to some physical checks and tests. Memory problems and confusion have many causes and aren't limited to the different types of dementia; the doctor therefore looks for specific physical signs that suggest these other diagnoses as well as for signs of the risk factors for dementia.

Physical examination

The physical examination consists of a top-to-toe check of the most relevant body systems that can show signs of diseases that may affect memory. With your circulation, brain and nervous system particularly in mind, the doctor

- ✔ Checks your blood pressure to make sure that it isn't high and examines your pulse for irregularities in its rhythm
- ✔ Carries out an examination of your heart and lungs with a stethoscope, looking particularly for signs of a heart murmur or poor lung capacity
- ✔ Examines your nervous system, including muscle power and tone, skin sensitivity and reflexes, because these may point to other diseases such as multiple sclerosis or strokes that can produce similar symptoms
- ✔ Prods your abdomen, concentrating particularly on checking for signs of liver disease

Memory tests

After a gruelling session of being questioned, prodded and poked, you may take the memory tests on a separate occasion. No doubt the traditional ten-minute GP consultation will have well and truly overrun and you'll be feeling quite wearied by it all anyway. If you're referred to an outpatient or hospital clinic, the tests will be more detailed, but most GPs will probably want to carry out one of two basic tests:

- ✔ Minicog
- ✔ GPcog (General Practitioner Assessment of Cognition)

These tests are very straightforward but are useful screening tools to give the doctor a good idea about whether you have a memory problem and therefore need more detailed cognitive tests.

The nearby sidebar provides an example of the sort of questions you're asked in a GPcog test.

Blood, urine and other tests

When the consultation's over, the doctor will probably send you away with some forms to take to your practice nurse so that you can have some blood tests and a urine sample sent to the laboratory at the local hospital for analysis. These tests are taken to rule out other possible conditions that can cause dementia-like symptoms but need a whole different type of treatment. In fact, many of them, unlike dementia itself, are treatable.

GPcog test

I will give you a name and address and would like you to repeat it back to me and then remember it, because I'll ask you to repeat it to me again at the end of the test:

✔ John Brown, 42 West Street, Kensington

✔ What is the date today? (Must be exact.)

✔ On the circle below, please mark in the numbers to indicate hours on a clock.

✔ Now draw in hands to show ten minutes past eleven o'clock (11:10).

✔ Can you tell me something that has happened in the news in the past week?

✔ What is the name and address I asked you to remember?

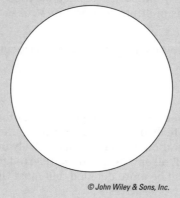

Samples are likely to be taken to check for the following:

✔ Signs of infection

✔ Anaemia

✔ Kidney or liver disease

✔ Diabetes

✔ Thyroid gland abnormalities

✔ Levels of vitamins such as B12 and folate

✔ Imbalances in minerals such as sodium, potassium and calcium

✔ Cystitis

You may also be asked to book in for an ECG (electrocardiogram, or heart tracing) if your GP noticed an abnormality when examining your heart, or a chest x-ray if your lungs didn't sound completely clear.

Working through the Next Stages of Investigation

Your GP will no doubt ask you to return to see her once all the tests are done, so that she can hopefully give you some kind of diagnosis or at least discuss a plan to take the investigations farther. If, from what she's seen, her assessment is that you're very unlikely to have dementia, she'll reassure you that all's well and offer to see you again should things deteriorate. If she's found another cause for your symptoms, such as anaemia or a urinary-tract infection, she'll start treatment for that.

If, however, your GP's investigations point towards a potential diagnosis of memory disorder, she'll refer you for more detailed tests. Initially, these are tests that she can arrange himself or with the help of specialist memory nurses who work in the community (or a clinic – not all areas have memory nurses). Your first port of call is likely to be the hospital x-ray department for a scan of your brain.

Undergoing brain scans

Unlike a car, where you simply lift up the bonnet and see what's going on in the engine underneath, access to the brain is, thankfully, restricted by the hard outer casing of the skull. Fortunately, advances in imaging techniques now allow doctors to take a peep at the brain's structures and some of its functions without having to physically lift the lid. And while these scans are only a piece of the diagnostic jigsaw and can give rogue results that are occasionally dismissed, they're a useful part of the investigation process.

Your doctor can choose one of four main types of scan. The choice is directed by what the doctor's looking for once she's analysed your other results and also, sadly, the financial availability of the different scans in the area of the country where you live.

CT scan

Computerised tomography (CT) scans are those most commonly available on the NHS. You lie in a large, doughnut-shaped scanner and completely painless x-rays penetrate your body tissues to different degrees depending on the amount of air and fluid they contain. A computer records the resulting images in thin slices from top to bottom.

These images are then analysed by a radiologist (a doctor who specialises in carrying out x-ray tests) to look for signs of disease. A scan of a normal brain has a classic appearance, so essentially the radiologist is checking your

CT scan for changes from normal. Different types of dementia have different patterns when looked at in a CT scanner; the radiologist looks for structural changes such as shrinkage of brain tissue in particular areas.

Occasionally, the radiologist injects dye into your bloodstream through a vein in the back of your hand to make some brain structures stand out more when scanned.

By and large, the CT scan is a simple and painless procedure that lasts up to half an hour, at most. If you're claustrophobic, you can be mildly sedated. The radiographer taking the images is in contact with you at all times through headphones.

MRI scan

Magnetic resonance imaging (MRI) scanners don't use x-ray radiation, like their CT scanner cousins, to capture images; instead they use magnetic fields and radio waves to build up a picture of your brain. An MRI scan shows blood flow in the brain better than a CT scan does, which can be useful if your doctor thinks you may have vascular dementia.

As a patient, you'll notice that you're in the scan (a tunnel) for a long time, usually around 45 minutes. The experience is very noisy; you will, however, be given headphones to try to drown out the mechanical din that these machines make.

Because MRI scanners are made with huge magnets, they're not suitable for people with metalwork surgically inserted into them, such as pacemakers or metal clips.

SPECT scan

Single-photon emission computed tomography (SPECT) scans are able to look in detail at how blood flows into tissues. These tests are most likely to be arranged by hospital specialists rather than GPs. To get this sort of information, you'll be injected with a liquid drug that contains a radiolabelled tracer. This tracer can then be detected as it flows through the brain, highlighting areas of greatest brain activity, which light up more brightly on the scan pictures, and those where blood flow, brain activity and therefore levels of tracer are much lower.

The different patterns of low activity in various areas of the brain can then help doctors to identify which type of dementia you have. So, for example, low blood flow is evident in the frontal lobes if you have fronto-temporal dementia, and in the middle of the temporal lobes, which are involved in memory, if you have Alzheimer's disease.

DAT scan

DAT is another type of scan that involves having an injection of a radioactive liquid into a vein. This substance is used to show up levels of a chemical transmitter in the brain called dopamine. Doctors use DAT scans to differentiate between Alzheimer's disease and the rarer Lewy body disease. They are only likely to be requested by hospital specialists and not by GPs.

Undergoing detailed psychological tests

A number of psychological tests are available, but Addenbrooke's cognitive examination (ACE-III) is particularly popular. Such tests may be carried out in your own doctor's surgery, but are more commonly administered by specialists. You can find an example of the ACE-III in Appendix B.

Being referred to a specialist

With medical history and examination completed, bloods taken, urine analysed, brain scanned and memory scores totted up, doctors will now be pretty certain about whether you have dementia.

If you have straightforward Alzheimer's disease or vascular dementia, you may well be looked after by your GP, with support from a dementia nurse in the community.

If, however, the diagnosis is still not clear cut, and it appears that you may have one of the less common types of dementia or an atypical version of one of the others, your GP may refer you on to see a specialist.

Identifying the specialists

Specialists work in a variety of settings around the country; the type of clinic you're referred to depends on where you live. You may be seen in a traditional hospital outpatient clinic, a specialist clinic in the community, a room in your GP's surgery or even in your own home.

Memory services are staffed by consultants from a variety of medical specialties, including medicine for the elderly, psychiatry and neurology, and the type of specialist you see varies across the UK. Regardless of their specialism, specialists will be well qualified to take your investigations forward and advise on appropriate treatment.

Most clinics are multidisciplinary nowadays, so rather than simply seeing a doctor, you may also be reviewed by a specialist memory nurse, community psychiatric nurse or psychologist too.

Considering what happens during an outpatient appointment

The specialist clinician will probably want to go back over the details of your medical history for herself, so if anything has cropped up since you saw your GP or you realise you forgot to tell her something, jot down the details so that you can tell the specialist. When the specialists are happy that they've got your story straight in their minds, they may also carry out another quick examination as well. Further examinations are more likely if you're seeing a neurologist or physician rather than a psychiatrist: these specialists will probably want to perform a thorough check on your nervous and circulatory systems.

After these initial assessments, you may be put through some of the more specialist scans, such as SPECT, which I describe earlier in this chapter, and maybe cognitive tests such as ACE-III too. Where these tests are carried out varies according to where in the UK you live. If these tests haven't been done prior to referral, your specialist is likely to want to make sure your battery of investigations is complete.

Sorting Out Follow-Up and an Ongoing Plan for Care

You now have a diagnosis, so what happens next? Unfortunately, no magic cure for dementia exists, whichever type you've been diagnosed with. Fortunately, however, some prescription medicines and various charities and social care organisations can help manage many of the more troublesome symptoms of the condition and help with long-term care needs.

You'll also need to address some important practical issues, such as

- Informing the DVLA about the diagnosis and the effect it has on your ability to drive and, possibly, your family if you're the only driver

- Planning for future financial management of your bank accounts, savings and insurance policies

- Establishing legal responsibility for ongoing care needs and timing of power of attorney

- Making a will if you don't already have one

- Deciding whether to continue with work and how to retire on the grounds of ill health when necessary

- Applying for benefits for your carers

Understanding what doctors can do

As with supporting you to take the first steps towards a diagnosis of dementia, your GP can also support you in the next steps after receiving your diagnosis. She has a handle not only on what the specialists have said about you, because she'll have received a letter detailing your diagnosis and management suggestions, but also on the most appropriate treatments to be tried and how to access the other help that's available.

Booking in to see your family doctor around two weeks after an appointment with the specialist is a good idea, because she'll be able to go through the details of the correspondence she's received from the hospital or clinic and also be able to translate any medical terms your specialist has used into plain English.

Don't be afraid to ask your GP anything, however daft you may think it sounds. GPs are there to help and are extremely willing to do so. And if your GP doesn't have an answer, she'll know whom to contact to get one.

Prescribe medication

Sadly, there's no 'pill for every ill', and that's particularly the case in relation to dementia. *But* pills are certainly available that can help improve the symptoms and, in some sufferers, even slow the disease's progression.

Your specialist or GP can advise about which medicines may help you. Unfortunately, she won't just be able to hand you a prescription, and some people will be disappointed to learn that the available medicines aren't suitable for them, not because of their cost to the NHS, but for clinical or safety reasons.

Reasons for not prescribing particular medicines include

- ✔ **Unsuitability for your type of dementia:** No drugs are licensed for all main types of dementia, and your doctor has to weigh up the risk of side effects you may experience with the potential benefits the drug may provide. If the drug isn't for your type of dementia, the possibilities for harm obviously come out on top.

- ✔ **Potential drug interactions with other medicines you're taking:** Drugs don't all get on with each other inside our bodies, and some interactions are potentially lethal. Thankfully, most aren't deadly, but they can still lead to some pretty nasty physical side effects. Other interactions may mean that a tablet you're already taking may not be so effective because of the addition of the new tablet or, conversely, may heighten its effects, making it potentially toxic.

✔ **Risk of making another medical condition you have much worse:** Very rarely do any pills act like magic bullets, targeting only the symptoms doctors want them to and not making mischief elsewhere in the body. That's because once you swallow a tablet or put on a patch, the drug's absorbed into your blood stream and whizzes all around your body. Consequently, if any other body tissues are sensitive to the chemical in your medicine, they'll be affected too. Aspirin provides a good example here: while preventing heart attacks and helping in vascular dementia, it can also cause stomach ulcers and potentially life-threatening haemorrhages in sensitive people.

Don't believe what you read in the tabloids. If your doctor won't prescribe you a particular medicine for your dementia, it's not because you're too old and she can't be bothered with you, or because it's too expensive and you're not worth it. Your GP probably won't prescribe it because she thinks it either won't help or, worse still, will make you ill.

All doctors practise according to the moral injunction to 'first do no harm', and that ethos guides all their decision making.

Identify suitable medication

Providing it's safe to do so and likely to help, your GP may prescribe a number of groups of medicines to help with your dementia and its knock-on effects. Below is a quick run-through of the types of drugs available (Chapter 7 covers them in more detail):

✔ **Drugs to treat dementia itself:** Four drugs are available at present (donepizil, rivastigmine, galantamine and memantine), all of which have been designed specifically to help Alzheimer's disease. Unfortunately, they provide no benefit for patients with fronto-temporal dementia or vascular dementia. These drugs are, however, sometimes used for people with a mixed diagnosis of Alzheimer's and vascular dementia, and can help a little in Lewy body disease. (Chapter 3 identifies the different forms of dementia.)

✔ **Drugs to protect against further deterioration:** Some Alzheimer's medicines have been shown to slow the progression of the disease for a while, and so are prescribed for this reason as well as to help with the symptoms of Alzheimer's. In vascular dementia, stopping further damage to blood vessels in the brain is very important, so doctors prescribe pills to make sure that your blood pressure and cholesterol are well controlled, and they may also give you pills such as aspirin to thin the blood and prevent blood clots from forming in your circulation.

✔ **Drugs to help with troublesome symptoms:** While not being designed to treat dementia specifically, a number of drugs nonetheless can help with the symptoms it can produce, which for some people can prove more disturbing than the condition itself. A common example of medicines in this category is antidepressants to help with anxiety and depression.

Provide monitoring and follow-up

Following diagnosis and the initiation of treatment, your doctors will want to keep an eye on you. They'll monitor the following:

✔ Whether your treatment's starting to work

✔ The development of any side effects from prescribed medication

✔ The state of your symptoms, to assess whether you're improving or are at least stable, or to pick up any deterioration in your condition that may require a change of management plan

✔ Your general physical health and the treatment of potential risk factors for your condition becoming worse

The timing of this follow-up varies between primary (GP surgery) and secondary (hospital) care. GPs are likely to see you more often than hospital doctors, who tend to review you quite infrequently and then discharge you back to your family doctor as soon as they're happy that your condition's stable.

You'll probably be seen by a variety of members of the healthcare team in both settings, and not just doctors. So be prepared for nurses of a variety of flavours (community nurses, practice nurses, specialist memory nurses) to keep an eye on you. They're often able to visit you at home to save trips to the surgery or clinic, and can consult the doctor for advice if any concerns are raised that are beyond their expertise (which will be very few!).

Accessing help from other therapists

At some point after your diagnosis, and this will vary from person to person, your doctor will probably enlist the help of a whole army of other clinicians working within the NHS to help with your symptoms and try to ensure that their impact on your life is kept to a minimum for as long as is humanly possible.

At first, if you're well and things are under control, you may not want or need any input. But if or when you do as the condition progresses over the years, it's good to know these therapists are out there. And while the NHS therapists can only be accessed by referral from your GP or specialist, a number of other professionals work privately, so you can get hold of them yourself.

Once again, not all these therapists will be available everywhere in the UK, but your GP will be able to tell you the best way to get help in your area.

NHS therapists

Your doctors can enlist the following therapists to help in your care:

- **Occupational therapists:** These therapists play a vital role in helping you maintain your ability to carry out everyday tasks from boiling a kettle to washing and bathing.

- **Physiotherapists:** These therapists play a vital role in helping you remain mobile.

- **Dieticians:** These therapists make sure that you're having a healthy, balanced diet and, if you have vascular dementia, keep you away from the high-cholesterol foods that can further fur up your arteries.

- **Counsellors/psychotherapists:** These therapists can help with psychological and emotional issues relating to the diagnosis of dementia; they also work with couples and carers to help resolve relationship difficulties and to offer support.

Chapter 13 looks in detail at the care and support that these therapists provide.

Complementary therapists

The so-called complementary therapies are rarely available on the NHS because they fall outside what's considered conventional medicine. They're also much less evidence based than medical treatments have to be in order to qualify for the use of government funds to promote their widespread use.

Some research has, however, shown that a few of these therapies do have some benefits in treating the symptoms of dementia. Although your doctor may be able to point you in the direction of a recommended therapist, bear in mind that you have to pay for any treatment you receive. The complementary therapies that do appear to help are

- Aromatherapy
- Bright light therapy
- Music therapy

Sorting out social care

Medical treatment is unfortunately pretty impotent in relation to dementia, thus the mainstay of help and support tends to come from social care. Social care is provided by local councils in conjunction with the NHS. Private companies and charities also offer valuable support to patients and their carers.

Your GP, specialist or memory nurse can tell you how to access these services, which in most cases involves you having a community care needs assessment.

Undergoing a community care needs assessment

Either you, a relative or a friend can arrange a community care needs assessment directly by contacting your local social services department or your GP, and other professionals involved in your care can request one on your behalf. Following the request, a care manager will contact you by phone or arrange for you to be visited at home.

The assessment can involve family members or friends, and looks at the following:

✔ Your living arrangements

✔ Your physical and mental limitations

✔ Specific worries experienced by you or your family

If you're found to be eligible for support, a written care plan is drawn up for you, usually by a social worker. This care plan, according to the NHS Choices website at www.nhs.uk, includes the following details:

✔ A list of your eligible care needs

✔ The goals or outcomes you want the plan to help you achieve

✔ Details of the services you'll receive and who's responsible for providing them

✔ Sources of funding for these services

✔ A risk assessment

✔ The name of the person responsible for implementing, monitoring and reviewing your care plan

✔ A review date on which to check that the care plan is meeting your needs

Checking out what's available

Apply for an assessment as soon as possible after you receive your diagnosis. Doing so means you'll find out early which services you're eligible for and also how to get extra help in the future as your condition progresses.

An extensive array of services is available, although again this can vary across the country, so don't struggle on unnecessarily. These services can include

✔ Home care, which can include assistance with shopping, cooking, cleaning, washing and dressing

✔ Meals on wheels

✔ Adaptations to your home such as hand rails, walk-in showers, access ramps and raised toilet seats

✔ Help taking medication

✔ Access to day centres and clubs

✔ Respite care

✔ Support filling in benefit forms and dealing with other money matters

Chapter 7

Medical Treatments in Dementia

· ·

In This Chapter

▶ Finding out about the drugs specifically designed to help the symptoms of dementia

▶ Looking at the medicines used to help depression and anxiety

▶ Knowing the side effects to watch out for when taking prescriptions

· ·

Medical science has made enormous advances over the past century and people now benefit from treatments for diseases affecting every system in the body, from infections to insomnia and headaches to heart disease. But still no pill exists for every ill, and for some conditions a cure seems to be some way off.

Unfortunately, dementia is in that category. No medicines on the market can see off all, or indeed any, of the underlying conditions that cause it. However, a handful of drugs slows down its progress and improves symptoms, if only temporarily. Alongside these specific medicines others can help manage some of the more difficult symptoms that dementia can throw up, such as sleeping difficulties, hallucinations and depression.

But because each person is unique, not all these medicines help all people, and in some cases although doctors prescribe medicines with the best of intentions, they can actually be harmful. This may be because they cause either already documented or unique side effects, or because they interact with pills the person is already taking.

So with these warnings in mind, this chapter takes a look at the drugs that are available to help with dementia and its troublesome symptoms, and discusses some of the unfortunate limitations they can have.

Identifying the Dementia Medicines

When you scan the chemist's shelves or browse in the supermarket's medicines section you see packet after packet of different pills designed to relieve all humanity's ailments. Usually, you see a dozen or so treatments for indigestion alone, a handful of headache remedies, boxes of different drugs to bung up diarrhoea and a similar number to treat bowels that need unblocking from constipation. Sadly, when it comes to dementia drugs the choice is nowhere near as extensive: in fact just four medicines are on offer (all of which are licensed for the treatment of Alzheimer's disease).

Dementia is at the forefront of government health policy, and it often makes headlines in the media. So hopefully investment into research by scientists and drug companies will continue, and the research will begin to bear fruit. But for now, here's a guide to what your specialist and GP have up their sleeves.

These medicines can help the symptoms of dementia, and particularly Alzheimer's disease, but they're not a cure for it.

The medicines that doctors prescribe for dementia have been designed to help with the cognitive symptoms and so improve memory and thought processes, and they can also help with mood and behaviour. They're available in a variety of formulations to help make them easy to take, and so come as pills, patches, liquids and soluble tablets.

As with all drugs, dementia medicines have a so-called *generic name*, which all manufacturers must use, and a *brand name*, which is the specific name a particular drug company gives to them. Here's an example with a well-known drug: ibuprofen is the generic name, and Nurofen is the brand name for the drug manufactured by Reckitt Benckiser. The more companies that make the drugs, the more brand names you find on the market.

Here are the four dementia drugs, with their generic names first, followed by their brand names in brackets:

- Donepezil (Aricept)
- Rivastigmine (Exelon, Kerstipon, Nimvastid)
- Galantamine (Acumor, Elmino, Galantex, Galsya, Gatalin, Lotprosin, Reminyl, Zeebral)
- Memantine (Ebixa)

Understanding How Dementia Drugs Work

The four medicines divide into two groups according to the different ways in which they work:

- **Acetylcholinesterase inhibitors:** Donepezil, rivastigmine, galantamine
- **Memantine:** A very small and lonely group of one!

Here's a quick guide to their different mechanisms.

Acetylcholinesterase inhibitors

Scientists have found that in Alzheimer's disease, the most common form of dementia, patients lose nerve cells in the brain that communicate with each other using a chemical neurotransmitter called *acetylcholine* (you can find more detail about the way these transmitters work in Chapter 4). As a result, communication is blocked and messages can't easily flow from one part of the brain to another. That means the person can't form new memories or recall them, and the other changes in mood, behaviour and thought processing that are characteristic of Alzheimer's disease occur.

The drugs in this group work by blocking the effect of an enzyme (*enzymes* are proteins in the body that promote chemical reactions) called acetylcholinesterase that breaks down acetylcholine. Acetylcholinesterase inhibitors therefore boost the level of acetylcholine once more and so improve symptoms.

Memantine

This drug works by affecting *glutamate*, one of the brain's chemical transmitters that's involved in the processes underlying learning and memory. It works by sticking to receptors on the walls of nerve cells called NMDA receptors (short for N methyl D aspartate receptors), which then unlocks channels in the cell wall that allow calcium to enter and work the biochemical magic needed to create memories.

Unfortunately, when the effects of Alzheimer's disease damage brain cells, these cells release much higher levels of glutamate than usual. The knock-on effect of this is a consequent rise in the amount of calcium flooding into cells. Because calcium is toxic to cells at high levels, the rise damages them even further.

Memantine sits on top of NMDA receptors (in technical parlance it's an *NMDA receptor agonist*) to stop the glutamate attaching and triggering this damaging chain of events. This, in turn, helps slow the progression of the Alzheimer's disease itself.

Knowing When to Start Taking the Drugs

The decision about when to start taking any medicine for dementia will be something you make jointly at the appointment with, and on the advice of, your specialist, although your GP may be the doctor who prints and signs the prescription itself. Your GP will also be involved in the ongoing monitoring of your progress while on the drug and in watching for any side effects, but you'll have periodic specialist reviews from time to time as well.

So you won't start on a drug until you have a formal diagnosis. Your GP certainly won't just give you some tablets, on the off chance that they could help your symptoms, on the first day you go to see him. After you have a diagnosis, though, you're likely to begin treatment straight away, as long as medical professionals think the drug is suitable and safe for you.

Timing can depend on the type of drug:

✓ **Acetylcholinesterase inhibitors:** National guidelines recommend that doctors give these medicines to people who have a diagnosis of mild to moderate Alzheimer's disease. Rivastigmine can also be used to treat symptoms in people who have Lewy body disease. Those who have mixed vascular dementia and Alzheimer's disease may also benefit.

Given the financial constraints on the National Health Service, doctors try the cheapest drug first, providing they think it's safe and will be effective. Prescriptions can be altered according to response to the treatment and any side effects you may have.

✓ **Memantine:** Doctors don't normally give memantine as a first resort, but reserve it for use in people who either don't get on with acetylcholinesterase inhibitors because of side effects or reactions, or who don't seem to respond to them. It's licensed for use in moderate to severe dementia, so is a logical next step if symptoms are severe. And some research evidence suggests that continuing the previous medicine while adding memantine on top can be beneficial.

Seeing How to Take the Medicines

Drugs to treat dementia symptoms come in a variety of formats. You get the lowest dose first and then your doctor can increase this if needed as time goes on. Table 7-1 is a guide to the formats, doses and administration of each of the four drugs.

Table 7-1		Taking Dementia Medicines	
	Formats	*Dose*	*Administration*
Donepezil	Ordinary and melt-in-the-mouth tablets	5 mg initially; increased after 1 month to 10 mg	The same each day; ideally at bedtime

	Formats	Dose	Administration
Rivastigmine	Tablets and patches	Tablets: 1.5 mg twice daily; can increase every 2 weeks in increments of 1.5 mg twice daily up to a maximum of 6 mg twice daily Patches: start at 4.6 mg every 24 hours; can be increased after 4 weeks to a usual dose of 9.5 mg every 24 hours on a 14 day rotation	Tablets: morning and evening Patches: applied to non-hairy skin on the upper arms, chest or back; must be changed to a different position at the same time every 24 hours
Galantamine	Ordinary and the more commonly used modified tablets; liquid	Ordinary tablets and liquid: 4 mg once daily for at least 7 days; then 4 mg twice daily for at least 4 weeks, reaching maximum of 8 mg twice daily Modified-release: start at 8 mg on alternate days for 7 days; then 8 mg once daily for 4 weeks, reaching maximum of 16 mg daily	Modified release tablets: morning Other preparations: same time each day; ideally morning and evening
Memantine	Tablets and liquid	Start on 5 mg once daily; can be increased weekly in 5-mg increments up to a maximum daily dose of 20 mg	Any time, but the same time each day

If you miss a dose, don't take two the next day to make up for it; simply take the next day's dose as normal.

You can take these medications for as long as they're giving you benefit. The Alzheimer's Society believes that around 40 to 70 per cent of people who take these drugs get some benefit from them and that this usually lasts for between 6 and 12 months, after which the effects of the dementia increase more slowly than would be expected without treatment.

Considering the Side Effects and Risks

No medicine comes without its possible side effects and, disappointingly, not all drugs are suitable for everyone who may benefit from them. Take into account the following points when taking dementia drugs.

Every box of pills that you get from the pharmacist comes with a leaflet stuffed inside it detailing all the possible side effects to look out for when taking your medication. Some lists are longer than others, and if you studied them in microscopic detail you'd never swallow anything your doctor ever prescribed, for fear that the cure was worse for you than the illness itself.

So although reading the leaflet is always a good idea, remember that the side effects listed are only possible and not definite, and the ones lower down the list are rare. Side effects are also less likely when you begin treatment at the lowest possible dose.

Side effects often wear off after a few days when you get used to taking the medication. So unless they're severe, persevere for a week or so to see whether the side effects settle.

Most people take the dementia drugs with very little trouble at all. The side effects of memantine are less likely to occur and generally less severe than for the acetylcholinesterase inhibitors. Here are some side effects to be aware of for both groups of drug:

- ✔ **Acetylcholinesterase inhibitors:** Loss of appetite, nausea, indigestion, stomach cramps and diarrhoea; headaches, dizziness, tiredness and insomnia; skin reactions from patches.

- ✔ **Memantine:** Headache, dizziness and tiredness; constipation; shortness of breath; raised blood pressure.

Who shouldn't take these drugs? Here's the lowdown:

- ✔ **Acetylcholinesterase inhibitors:** Other than breast-feeding mums (who very rarely develop dementia), no groups of people exist who absolutely shouldn't take these drugs. Doctors do, however, prescribe them with caution to people with established heart, liver, lung or kidney disease, anyone who has a medical history of having fits and pregnant women.

- ✔ **Memantine:** Not ideal for pregnant women or if you have epilepsy. Also avoid if you have raised blood pressure; heart, kidney or liver problems; or recently you had a heart attack.

Looking at Other Drugs That Help Alleviate Symptoms

Doctors often prescribe medicines designed for other conditions to help deal with some of the troublesome symptoms that dementia can cause. These other drugs have their downsides, and not all are suitable for all four main types of dementia. The following sections tell you what you need to know.

Antidepressant drugs

Depression is extremely common in society as a whole and people with dementia frequently suffer from it. Its symptoms include

- ✔ Irritability
- ✔ Loss of interest in doing things
- ✔ Low mood
- ✔ Poor concentration and memory
- ✔ Poor sleep and appetite
- ✔ Tearfulness
- ✔ Thoughts of death and perhaps even suicide

Depression can also provoke feelings of anxiety and worry.

Dementia plus depression is an unfortunate double whammy that can make the symptoms of the dementia worsen more quickly than in normal disease progression. Treating the depression can therefore make a big difference all round to the person's wellbeing.

Understanding how antidepressants work

Antidepressant tablets increase the levels of neurotransmitters in the brain that are thought to dip when you have depression. The main transmitters affected are serotonin and noradrenaline. The pills don't give a fake dose of these neurotransmitters but give your own depleted levels a boost and increase the number of receptors to them to make them more effective.

Most people find that antidepressants begin to help after a couple of weeks, during which time any side effects come and go. You'll be on them for between four to six months in total and then weaned off them. They're not addictive.

Knowing when doctors prescribe antidepressants

Your GP or specialist will suggest you start these medicines if he senses you have a significant case of depression. He usually goes on symptoms alone, but won't rush for the prescription pad the minute you say you've been down in the dumps for a few days.

Alongside their usefulness in treating depression, antidepressants can help with symptoms of severe anxiety and worry too. And evidence suggests that in dementia particularly they can help reduce agitation and also improve motivation if you find you've lost interest in life.

Being aware of the side effects and risks

These depend on the type of medication used. Doctors most commonly prescribe the SSRIs (selective serotonin reuptake inhibitors) for dementia patients, and their main possible side effects are

- ✔ Nausea, indigestion, stomach ache, diarrhoea, loss of appetite and constipation
- ✔ Headaches, tiredness and loss of sexual desire

Doctors use them cautiously in people with epilepsy, heart disease, diabetes and any history of bleeding into the bowel. They can also interact with some strong painkillers such as tramadol.

Sleeping tablets

Disturbed sleep patterns are, unfortunately, a common symptom of dementia, and a serious one. The person with dementia is at risk of falls at night, not to mention daytime exhaustion, and carers are at risk of never getting any sleep themselves. The difficulty can be either with dropping off in the first place or waking frequently through the night. And some unlucky people struggle with a bit of both.

Understanding how sleeping tablets work

Two main groups of antidepressant drugs exist, and each has a slightly different chemical make-up:

- ✔ Benzodiazepines
- ✔ Z drugs (so-called because their names all start with the letter Z)

Both work by increasing the level of the neurotransmitter GABA (gamma-aminobutyric acid) in the brain. This in turn increases drowsiness and triggers sleep.

Doctors sometimes prescribe other medicines that aren't officially sleeping tablets but cause sleepiness as a side effect. Some of these are antidepressants, such as trazodone, dosulepin and amitriptyline. Others are antihistamines, such as hydroxyzine.

Finally, some people over the age of 55 may be prescribed melatonin. This is a naturally occurring hormone produced in the brain that's involved in sleep–wake cycles and the regulation of the body clock. A dose of this also triggers sleep.

Knowing when doctors prescribe sleeping tablets

Sleeping pills are a last resort for treating sleep disturbances. So doctors only consider prescribing them when patients have tried and failed to improve sleep with simple measures like increasing daytime activity, cutting down on napping, reducing daily caffeine intake and taking *bright-light therapy* (which involves using light boxes to reinforce a person's sense of night and day; for more detail see Chapter 8).

Being aware of the side effects and risks

Sleeping pills are notoriously addictive and as a result no one should take them for more than two weeks at a time. So they're not a long-term solution to night-time problems.

The drowsiness sleeping tablets cause can make incontinence and 'accidents' with toileting more likely and put people in danger of having falls because of unsteadiness. They can also affect breathing, so shouldn't be given to people with lung diseases or sleep apnoea.

Antipsychotic drugs

These medicines were initially developed to treat people who suffer with severe mental health conditions like schizophrenia. They were the first pills to help rid patients of disturbing symptoms like delusional ideas, paranoia and hallucinations, and enabled sufferers to live more normal lives in the community rather than being admitted into asylums to be forgotten about.

As a result of their actions, antipsychotics can help with hallucinations and delusions in dementia and settle aggression and agitation (the drug risperidone is licensed to do just that).

Understanding how antipsychotic drugs work

Two main groups of antipsychotic medications exist, separated chronologically into older antipsychotics (chlorpromazine and haloperidol are examples) and newer ones (like risperidone, amisulpride and olanzapine). The newer drugs, developed since the 1970s, have fewer side effects than those made earlier.

Antipsychotics work on neurotransmitters. They affect serotonin, noradrenaline and acetylcholine, but the majority of their action comes from their particular role in blocking dopamine.

Knowing when doctors prescribe antipsychotics

Doctors keep these drugs in reserve and use them only when people have really serious and distressing behavioural or psychological symptoms. Although they help about 50 per cent of people who take them, doctors don't prescribe them for more than 12 weeks and they monitor patients closely throughout for severe side effects.

Why do drugs have side effects?

All drugs can have potential side effects because in essence when you take a medicine you're putting a dose of an unfamiliar chemical into your body that has the potential to disagree with you. Thankfully, given the number of prescriptions issued by doctors each year, very few side effects turn out to be serious. But even the mildest and most temporary (as most of them are) can be quite a nuisance.

People experience side effects for a variety of reasons, some to do with individual constitutions and some to do with the chemical make-up of the drugs themselves.

Here are some constitutional reasons:

- **Allergy:** These can cause the most severe side effects and can potentially be life threatening.

- **Intolerance:** This is milder than an allergy but can still cause the body to react against the medication. Intolerance usually leads to stomach upsets, bowel trouble or headaches.

- **Different rates of drug metabolism:** Some enzymes in the body are protein molecules that help break down and dispose of anything you take into your body, from pills to puddings. Some people have less effective systems than others, which means

that doses of medicines may end up being higher than they need to be, which causes side effects.

- **Other medical conditions:** Breakdown in the liver and excretion by the kidneys removes drugs from the body. If these organs are working below par, drug levels in the bodies are higher than needed.

- **Age:** As you get older the body's methods of breaking down and removing drugs become less efficient.

Sometimes side effects are down to the drugs:

- **Collateral damage:** The drugs in this chapter work on receptors for chemical transmitters on cells in the bodies (in the case of dementia, on nerve cells in the brain). Unfortunately, these receptors aren't just on the cells that you want to affect; they're on cells all over the body. And as drugs travel throughout the blood stream, they affect these receptors wherever they find them. This causes unwanted effects.

- **Interactions:** Drugs don't all get on with each other, and when you take more than one medicine they may interact with each other, causing side effects.

Being aware of the side effects and risks

The side effects of antipsychotics are quite wide ranging because the drugs affect so many different neurotransmitters in the brain. Dopamine is involved in movement (people with Parkinson's disease have low levels in their brains) and so shakiness and unsteadiness are common side effects, along with a corresponding greater risk of having a fall. Antipsychotics can also cause headaches, tiredness and stomach upsets.

Doctors use antipsychotics with caution in people with heart disease and never give them to people with Lewy body disease. Half of people with this condition have a severe sensitivity to antipsychotics that can worsen symptoms and even, in some cases, be fatal.

Chapter 8

Considering Non-Medical Treatment

*M*any treatments are touted for dementia that aren't dished out on a green prescription pad by the doctor. Known variously as complementary or alternative therapies (see the nearby sidebar), some are more valid and useful than others! Unfortunately, a lot of nonsense is out there. Tap 'alternative medicine + dementia' into a search engine and you'll be introduced to potential treatment cocktails that seem more like something dreamed up by JK Rowling for a potions class than medicines to treat a neurodegenerative brain disorder.

I regularly meet patients, however, who swear that this or that herbal tincture or dietary supplement has had a genuinely positive effect on the cognitive functions of someone they know. And I'm a liberal enough doctor not to heavy-handedly dissuade anyone from trying a treatment that may work for her, even if the evidence for its efficacy is less than flimsy (unless the treatment is obviously known to be downright dangerous).

In this chapter I provide an open-minded but honest appraisal of the most commonly cited complementary therapies advertised as treatments for the symptoms of dementia. Some of these utilise herbs or vitamins, or cocktails of the two, while others are more physical, interactive therapies.

The scientific evidence for the effectiveness of many complementary treatments is either non-existent or at least not as robust as that for prescription medicines. And while I would never deter anyone from trying something as long as it was safe, I don't believe it's safe to stick exclusively to herbal or homoeopathic remedies and the like at the expense of treatments that a doctor recommends, because I know they'll help.

Vitamins and Herbal Remedies

Plants, herbs and the vitamins they contain have been used as remedies for human ailments for millennia. And even in the 21st century, there's still a large market for these more natural pharmaceuticals. A few of these are touted as treatments for the symptoms of dementia, and the following sections cover some of the most frequently mentioned herbal remedies with details of where they come from, what they are supposed to do and a review of their effectiveness.

Just because a treatment is 'natural' doesn't mean that it's without possible side effects and may not interact with other medicines you're on.

Gingko biloba

When it comes to herbal remedies famed for their healing properties in dementia – in fact, all the complementary therapies put together – *gingko biloba* is probably the most lauded. It crops up so often when you search on the Internet that it can almost be considered a mainstream treatment.

This plant extract comes from the gingko or maidenhair tree, which is commonly called a 'living fossil' because it's been a feature of the earth's landscape since it shared it with the dinosaurs; their fossilised ancestors are commonly found in rocks from the Jurassic and Cretaceous periods. Gingko trees can grow all over the world but are most commonly found in China and Japan. The oldest known specimen was 3,500 years old.

Active ingredients

The leaves of the tree are believed to have medicinal properties and, when analysed scientifically, have been found to contain two main groups of active chemicals: flavonoids and terpenoids. *Flavonoids* have antioxidant properties and are thought to have most effect on the nervous system; *terpenoids* improve blood flow by dilating blood vessels and stopping platelets from sticking to each other to form blood clots within the body.

The double action of protecting brain cells and improving blood supply is thought to explain gingko's therapeutic effects. As a result, gingko is suggested to help people with both Alzheimer's disease and vascular dementia by

- ✔ Improving their cognitive functions, particularly memory
- ✔ Reducing their chance of developing mood changes, especially depression
- ✔ Improving their ability to carry out everyday tasks and to socialise with other people

Free radicals

Contrary to the sound of the name, *free radicals* have nothing whatsoever to do with underground resistance movements in the Second World War; nor are they closet revolutionaries. Instead, they're atoms or groups of atoms with a spare unpaired electron (electrons are happiest hanging out in pairs) that makes them extremely unstable and reactive. Inside the human body, these free radicals go 'looking' for another electron with which to create a pair, and they do so by bumping into other molecules and stealing electrons from them. The burgled molecule then becomes a free radical itself and, in turn, bumps into another molecule – and so on.

In the human body, these free radicals can damage the structure of cells, the components inside cells and even the genetic material (DNA) itself. This damage stops the cells from working normally and can lead to disease. In dementia, damage to brain cells is what causes the problem.

Free radicals are naturally generated by chemical reactions that take place inside us all the time. However, environmental factors can also produce free radicals – air pollution and inhaled cigarette smoke being the main culprits.

Thankfully, our bodies produce natural antidotes to these free radicals, called *antioxidants*. These are stable molecules that can donate an electron to a free radical and then neutralise it. The body's normal metabolic processes produce antioxidants in an attempt to prevent possible damage.

Many foods also contain antioxidants, which is why you're encouraged to eat five portions of fruit and veg a day (and why herbal and vitamin-based therapies are advocated). To add antioxidants to your diet, put the following fruit and vegetables on your weekly shopping list:

- ✔ Berries such as strawberries, blackberries, blueberries and raspberries

- ✔ Fruits like grapes, cherries, plums, bananas, kiwis and pineapples

- ✔ Vegetables, including kale, red cabbage, broccoli, asparagus, potatoes and tomatoes

- ✔ Nuts such as pistachios, walnuts, pecans and hazelnuts

Side effects

Gingko seems to be almost side-effect free. However, in addition to the usual minor stomach upsets, skin rashes, dizziness and headaches that can accompany ingestion of any medication, it has one notable side effect.

Gingko inhibits the stickiness of platelets, and thus needs to be discontinued a couple of days before surgery to avoid the risk of haemorrhage.

Gingko is also known to interact with a number of prescription medicines:

- ✔ **Anticonvulsants:** The effectiveness of anticonvulsants, used to treat epilepsy, may be reduced by gingko, increasing the risk of seizures. The carbamazepine and sodium valproate in anticonvulsants are highly likely to interact with gingko in this way.

✔ **Antidepressants:** Selective serotonin reuptake inhibitors (SSRIs – a group that includes citalopram, sertraline, fluoxetine and paroxetine) can interact with gingko and set off *serotonin syndrome*, the symptoms of which include high blood pressure, a racing heart, excessive sweating, a tremor, muscle rigidity, increased reflexes, anxiety, agitation and potentially coma. It's best avoided!

✔ **Antihypertensives:** Because it dilates the blood vessels, gingko can cause the blood pressure to drop. For people already on medication to treat hypertension, this fall can be enormous.

✔ **Anticoagulants:** The effects of all medicines used to thin the blood can be magnified by the similar effects of gingko, if the treatments are taken together. Particular care should be taken by people on warfarin, aspirin or clopidogrel.

Evidence

Gingko actually seems to help. Research conducted in Germany with over 2,000 patients, the results of which were published in 2010, demonstrated definite benefits accruing from treating symptoms of dementia with gingko extract over those of a placebo.

Comparisons of the effects of gingko versus those of approved dementia medicines such as rivastigmine have, however, not been so positive – the pharmaceuticals come out on top. And while a 20-year study published in 2013 by a team from Bordeaux found that gingko reduced expected cognitive decline in healthy older people, other researchers have found that it has no actual protective benefit in reducing the occurrence of dementia itself.

Gingko is thus by no means a miracle drug and no substitute for prescription medicines for dementia. However, for those not taking any of the medicines that may interact negatively with it, gingko may be well worth a shot.

Vitamin E

The number of people delving into Mother Nature's medicine chest to look for more 'organic' ways to treat disease has resulted in a huge market for vitamin supplements. Never-ending combinations of vitamins are advertised as cure-alls for everything from the common cold to arthritis. In relation to dementia, vitamin E is supposed to work wonders.

Like all vitamins, vitamin E is found naturally in plant extracts, fruit and vegetables. Ideally, you'll get all the vitamins you need from your diet rather than popping them in pill form. Natural sources of vitamin E include

✔ Sunflower and olive oil

✔ Almonds and hazelnuts

 ✔ Kiwi fruit, mangoes, tomatoes

 ✔ Pumpkins, turnips, avocados, asparagus, sweet potatoes

 ✔ Fish and shellfish

With a list that good and wholesome, no wonder vitamin E is thought to do some good.

Vitamin E also has a role in protecting the outer layer of human cells, called the membrane, which in turn protects and maintains the normal function of cells themselves.

Active ingredient

As with gingko, antioxidants are suggested to be the active ingredient in vitamin E.

Side effects

Unfortunately, just because something is natural and found in something as tasty as kiwi fruit, it doesn't mean that it can't cause unpleasant side effects when industrially concentrated into a pill. The most frequently reported problems are sickness and diarrhoea, and muscle weakness.

Vitamin E can also interact with prescription medicines designed to thin the blood, such as warfarin and clopidogrel, increasing the risk of abnormal bleeding and bruising. Even worse, some research evidence shows that prolonged intake of high doses of vitamin E can actually increase your risk of death.

Evidence

Much of the research on the effects of vitamin E has been conducted with animals. A paper published in the *Journal of the American Medical Association* (*JAMA*) in early 2014 suggests, however, that the benefits accruing from vitamin E supplements may be genuine. The research team carried out a randomised controlled trial whereby 613 participants received doses of vitamin E, the dementia drug memantine, vitamin E plus memantine or an inactive placebo. The results showed that, while none of these treatments were effective in slowing down cognitive function itself, people's ability to carry out their usual daily activities declined more slowly when they took vitamin E than if they took a placebo. Taking memantine together with vitamin E provided no extra benefit.

Unfortunately, while this finding suggests a modest but genuine benefit from taking vitamin E, uncertainty still remains regarding the safety of taking the high doses used in the study for a sustained period of time.

While the jury's out, sticking to other medicines is probably the best advice for now.

Huperzine A

Huperzine A has been around for centuries as a staple ingredient of Chinese medicine. It's used to help memory and reduce inflammation. Native to India and southeast Asia, huperzine A is an extract from the fir clubmoss plant *Huperzia serrata*.

Active ingredient

Huperzine A is a chemical with similar anticholinesterase action to prescription drugs such as donepezil and rivastigmine. *Anticholinesterase* is an enzyme that breaks down the nerve transmitter acetylcholine, which is important for many mental functions, including memory. The huperzine A sticks to the anticholinesterase, which stops it attaching to acetylcholine and breaking it down. The acetylcholine level therefore rises, giving it more chance to boost brain function.

Side effects

Huperzine A does have a few unpleasant side effects in susceptible people. The commonest are

- Chest and throat tightness
- Slower heart rate
- Stomach upset (pain, loose bowels, nausea)
- Insomnia

Huperzine A isn't recommended for use with children or pregnant women because not enough is known about its safety in these groups. It may also potentially interact with prescribed medication for dementia, so shouldn't be taken alongside it. Treatments for the eye disease glaucoma may work less effectively as a result of taking huperzine A, obviously making that disease worse as a result.

Evidence

Early small-scale studies have shown some promise, with improvements in people's memory and reductions in the level of disability their dementia causes. But so far too little convincing evidence exists to justify huperzine A being recommended as a first-line treatment, especially because drugs are already available that not only work in the same way but have also been tested for safety.

Alternative or complementary therapies

These two terms are often used interchangeably in relation to non-medical treatments. A variety of alternative practitioners exist, some of whom belong to their own professional bodies, such as osteopaths, homoeopaths and herbalists, while some don't. To ensure that you use a reputable therapist, check whether the person is on the register of the Complementary and Natural Healthcare Council (CNHC) (www.cnhc.org.uk). This body registers only practitioners who conform to a strict code of conduct, performance and ethics.

You'll notice that the CNHC uses the term 'complementary' rather than 'alternative' to describe its therapies, and I think that's an important distinction, because while many of these treatments can complement those of registered medical practitioners, they shouldn't be seen as substitutes or alternatives. Treatments recommended and prescribed by doctors and other members of the healthcare team have been subjected to stringent testing and analysis to ensure their safety and effectiveness. They may have side effects, but are nonetheless safe to use.

VITACOG

VITACOG is the name given to a cocktail of B-group vitamins (B6, B12 and folic acid) developed by a team at Oxford University to see whether it could help put the brakes on the rate of cognitive decline in people with dementia. It's generated a fair amount of media coverage and excitement.

In the study, the ingredients were blended by the researchers, but the B vitamins used are found naturally as follows:

- ✔ **B6:** Poultry, pork, fish, cereals, rice, eggs, milk, potatoes, soya, vegetables
- ✔ **B12:** Meat, fish, milk, eggs, cheese, fortified breakfast cereals
- ✔ **Folic acid:** Broccoli, Brussels sprouts, spinach, peas, chickpeas, fortified cereals, liver

Active ingredients

The vitamins themselves are the active ingredients in VITACOG. They work by reducing the levels of an amino acid called *homocysteine*. As people age, the homocysteine level in the body rises, causing damage to nerve cells in the brain and leading to their eventual death. Death of these cells causes brain shrinkage and a decline in cognitive function.

The B vitamins in VITACOG are known to reduce homocysteine levels and thus act to protect the brain from this potential damage.

Side effects

Side effects from VITACOG are minimal, but interactions with iron tablets and anticoagulant therapy are possible.

Evidence

So far, treating dementia with B vitamins shows encouraging results. The participants in the Oxford University study did demonstrate reduced brain shrinkage as a result of lowering their homocysteine levels, but it's too early to tell whether this physical improvement in brain structure improves symptoms of established dementia or actually holds off its development altogether. Research continues.

Medical Foods

Medical foods developed to help fight dementia, and particularly Alzheimer's disease, have received extensive media coverage. Described as 'miracle milk-shakes', two such products are Souvenaid and Axona.

The two drinks contain different combinations of nutrients designed to reduce damage to brain cells and therefore improve cognitive functioning.

The maker of Souvenaid, Nutricia, lists the following among the product's ingredients:

- Omega 3 fish oils
- Phospholipids
- Choline
- Folic acid and vitamins B6, B12, C and E
- Selenium

This combination is designed to help nerve cells in the brains of people with Alzheimer's disease make new connections (called synapses) and, as a result, repair the damage caused by the disease and thus reduce its symptoms.

In contrast to the multiple constituent ingredients in Souvenaid, Axona effectively has just one – caprylic triglyceride – which is derived from coconut oil. It's designed to provide the brains of people with Alzheimer's with a new form of energy when their ability to use the glucose the brain cells normally rely on for doing so is reduced.

The milkshakes both produce low-level side effects, the main symptoms being upset bowels, nausea and a bit of flatulence. Axona should also be used with caution by people with poorly controlled diabetes.

In terms of evidence, some small-scale studies have revealed some improvement in people with mild dementia as a result of using Souvenaid and Axona. But these products are very expensive and aren't available on prescription, so the small potential benefit is probably outweighed by the financial cost.

Aromatherapy

While the term aromatherapy is relatively modern, the use of aromatic oils as a treatment for illness certainly isn't. Records of the use of aromatic oils date as far back as 3000 BC, and who knows for how long people used this type of therapy before they bothered recording that they were doing so? Many references are made to the use of aromatic oils in Egyptian, Greek and Roman medicine. Today, around 400 different essential oils are in frequent use.

The oils used in aromatherapy are extracted from a wide variety of species, each one believed to have its own particular effect on the mind and body. Of the hundreds of oils available, the following are thought to help in dementia:

- ✔ Basil
- ✔ Chamomile
- ✔ Coriander
- ✔ Lavender
- ✔ Lemon and lemon balm
- ✔ Neroli

Application

Aromatherapists work in a holistic way with their clients. First they discuss the client's medical history and the particular symptoms causing concern, and then they decide which oil or combination of oils to use.

The aromatherapy oils can then be delivered to people's bodies in a number of different ways:

- ✔ **Massage:** Applying directly to the skin.
- ✔ **Baths:** Adding a few drops to the water, both to make direct contact with the skin and for the person to inhale the steam.
- ✔ **Inhalations and vaporisers:** Providing the oil in the form of a smoke-like vapour, often using candles.
- ✔ **Compresses:** Applying directly to the site of an injury or localised pain.

Considering how it works

Aromatherapists believe that oil molecules enter the body through the skin and the lining of the lungs and then work their way into the blood stream. From there, the oil molecules travel around the body to perform their healing duties by interacting with hormones and other biochemicals.

Researchers, however, aren't yet sure about the mechanisms at work during aromatherapy. The commonest theory is that the effect of the scents is achieved via the smell (olfactory) receptors in the nose, which are linked by nerve pathways to the areas in the brain involved in memory and emotion. Once stimulated, these areas of the brain in the limbic system (most commonly the amygdala and hippocampus) release yet more chemicals in the patient's body, leading to feelings of relaxation and calm. The theory seems to make sense.

Unfortunately, the evidence is inconclusive. However, many researchers have found small improvements in levels of agitation and distress – two of the main behavioural symptoms of dementia – as a result of aromatherapy, and so it's certainly worth a try.

Reminiscence Therapy

Chatting to friends and family about happy times shared in the past generally makes us feel good inside. Remembering the late 1970s and 1980s, or better still seeing TV clips or hearing songs from that era, does it for me. I particularly love reminiscing about anything to do with the mod revival of 1980: the Harrington jackets covered with badges, slim ties, straight-legged trousers and tassled loafer shoes. And I'm transported back to those happy times whenever I hear a song by Madness or the Specials on the radio, or they show clips of *Top of the Pops* appearances of The Jam on television.

Reminiscence therapy aims to tap into intact fond memories. The sights, sounds, tastes and even smells of a cherished past can help to improve life for someone whose present makes no sense and is quite a scary place to inhabit. In fact, evidence shows that this type of therapy not only improves the mood of someone with dementia but also has a positive effect on general wellbeing and maintaining relationships with carers, friends and family members. And it can improve some aspects of cognitive function too.

Not all reminiscences are happy or positive. Some prompts may remind a person of past hurt or trauma. Reminiscence therapy may bring back memories of people the person has lost, for example, and the grief she experiences may be as vivid as if the person has just died. These bad memories must be dealt with sensitively and not ignored in the hope that they'll go away on their own. Let the person with dementia talk about her feelings and have a good cry if she needs to.

Don't assume that everyone wants to spend time looking at their past. Engagement in reminiscence therapy must be voluntary if it's to be beneficial.

Reminiscence therapy holds as many possibilities as your imagination can produce. You can carry out one-to-one or group sessions, whichever seem most appropriate. Reminiscence therapy is suitable in a variety of settings, such as people's home, day centres, care homes and even hospital.

You can use a whole range of media, from photos and cine films to books, records and old magazines, and even favourite foods and drinks. Working on a scrapbook of things to refer back to time and again is a nice idea.

Here are a few suggestions for appealing to each of the senses:

- ✔ **Sound:** Most of us have a favourite song, individual piece of music or even whole genre, such as jazz or dance hall tunes, which we like to listen to because the music takes us to a place in our heads that nothing else can reach. Maybe a particular song reminds us of a first date, the sensation of falling in love, the first dance at our wedding or simply the soundtrack of a favourite film.

  Reminiscing about music, playing it again and talking about how it affects someone can be a useful part of reminiscence therapy. It can lead on to discussions about the people, places and times that made it special.

- ✔ **Touch:** Holding favourite items of jewellery or cherished ornaments can lead into some interesting conversations about where they came from and the special memories they evoke. Old clothing, like a jumper or fur coat, can also trigger such memories. Medals and trophies can be particularly good tools for reminiscence – although they may bring back sad as well as happy memories.

- ✔ **Sight:** Looking at old family photo albums or cine films can be a good start here. Books of photographs of someone's home town, newsreels of historic events and favourite old films can all trigger reminiscences.

- ✔ **Taste and smell:** Food and drink can also be shared and used to trigger thoughts of people and places. You could involve the person with dementia in cooking a favourite meal, or set up a restaurant scene and encourage a group of participants to chat and share memories of meals abroad or with love ones.

Quizzes and sing-alongs to old favourites can also be a great way to encourage people to communicate and connect with each other. The more fun, the better.

Music Therapy

Music has the power to move us. The melody, words or context can inspire joy or deep sorrow. Music can provide very personal experiences: songs can both move me to tears and make me jump around the bedroom yelling lyrics into a hairbrush or strumming the life out of an air guitar. Music can also have a powerful effect on groups of people in congregations and audiences, from the sacred connections formed while singing hymns in church to the equally spiritual experience of singing along with a band in a field at a music festival, arms raised, cigarette lighters aglow.

Music therapy uses these emotional responses to try to improve a person's sense of wellbeing through both listening to and joining in with voices or instruments.

Music and the brain

Music was probably a feature of human civilisation from the very start. Music is ubiquitous; every culture has a musical tradition. It's easy to imagine our earliest ancestors in Africa's Rift Valley singing and playing instruments while hanging out together around the camp fire. In fact, archaeologists have found flutes carved from animal bones and horns at sites in Germany dating back at least 35,000 years. While not quite providing evidence all the way back to our human origins, this find nonetheless demonstrates that music has been important enough to have been passed on to generation after generation of our species. Given that it has no obvious value in terms of survival, why has music become so pervasive in human society?

Neuroscientist Robert Zatorre from McGill University in Montreal, Canada, leads a research team trying to answer that question. Using modern scanning techniques, the team have shown that when people experience a spine-tingling feeling when listening to a favourite tune, a corresponding release of the chemical neurotransmitter dopamine occurs in a part of the brain called the striatum. The brain has similar responses to food and sex in this region, and it's artificially stimulated by some addictive drugs like cocaine.

The effect of music on the brain is a fascinating and evolving area of research. But the fact that it leads to an emotional reward no doubt goes some way to explaining why it touches most of us so profoundly. Add this to the discovery by researchers in Berlin that musical memories are stored differently to other memories and are therefore still retrievable by people with dementia, and it's easy to see how listening to music and singing along may be therapeutic.

How music helps

I encountered the most moving example of the effectiveness of music to reach someone whose brain is profoundly affected by dementia at a conference in 2013 on the role of the voice in medicine. Attendees were shown a video clip of an 80-year-old woman with Alzheimer's disease; I'll call her Marjorie.

Marjorie was in the advanced stages of the disease, was completely dependent on others for care, did not mix with fellow residents in the care home where she lived and had not spoken a word to anyone for weeks. But she did let the music therapist into her room when he visited. The film clip the therapist showed us featured him in Marjorie's room as he strummed his guitar, playing a variety of different tunes that she may have known when she was younger. And as the clip went on, we saw her open her mouth and join in. She wasn't singing the recognised words, and she was a few octaves out of tune, but she was making sounds in time with the music. For the first time in an absolute age, she was communicating with another human being. We watched her response to the music in amazement, and by the end of the film there was barely a dry eye in the audience. The music had touched her somewhere far deeper than the areas of her brain that the Alzheimer's had destroyed, and once again Marjorie had a voice. She visibly came alive in front of us.

At the end of the clip, we saw her stop singing and once again go quiet. They were the last sounds anyone heard her utter, because she sadly died a short while later.

Two main types of therapy are available:

- ✔ **Receptive therapy:** The therapist plays and sings and the audience simply listens.
- ✔ **Active therapy:** People are encouraged to join in singing and playing simple instruments.

Effectiveness

Having seen the effect of music on Marjorie, I need little convincing that music therapy works in ways that other treatments for dementia cannot in terms of connecting with people. But a wealth of research evidence also backs up anecdotal examples such as Marjorie's. And although these studies are often small scale and therefore not able to draw the hard-and-fast conclusions of large studies, plenty of evidence suggests that in moderate to severe dementia music therapy

- ✔ Can reduce the occurrence and severity of troublesome behavioural problems
- ✔ Reduces the symptoms of anxiety and depression
- ✔ Improves communication and social functioning
- ✔ Reduces blood pressure

Music therapy is also, of course, free from side effects and doesn't interact with other forms of treatment. It's definitely worth a try.

Reality Orientation

We all know the feeling of disorientation that occurs when waking up in a strange bed – at a friend's house, in a hotel, in a holiday cottage. You've just come out of a deep sleep and come to in a lovely warm bed, just like your own, but the walls are a different colour, the pictures are unfamiliar and the alarm clock isn't where it should be. In fact, neither is the bedside table it should be sitting on.

Thankfully, it doesn't take long to realise where you are, the confusion dissipates and you start to become familiar with your new surroundings. But imagine how disorientating this confusion can be for someone with dementia. You're not sure where you are or what day it is – and you may experience that sensation every morning on awakening. And throughout the day, during all activities, you may not recognise your surroundings or the person sitting next to you. You can understand why people with dementia are often very agitated and distressed.

Reality orientation aims to reduce confusion by giving a person with dementia a better sense of people, place and time. It reinforces people's awareness of who they are, whom they're with, where they are, and the date and time.

You can reinforce someone's sense of reality by

- ✔ Displaying on a board the day, date, time of next meal and even weather. You must remember to change it every day!
- ✔ Mounting large wall clocks in each room
- ✔ Buying daily newspapers (and putting old ones in the recycling bin)

✔ Putting signs on each door to identify the purpose of each room

✔ Making sure that everyone wears name badges, if the person is in a care home

✔ Actively discussing current events, frequently using the person's name in conversation and referring to the day of the week as often as possible

Risks and benefits

Research has shown that reality orientation can produce positive results, particularly when used alongside dementia medication. A study published in the *British Journal of Psychiatry* in 2005, for example, showed improvement in memory and other cognitive test scores in participants experiencing reality orientation therapy over a 25-week period compared to those receiving pills only. And other studies have found that reality orientation also has a positive effect on people's ability to socially interact with others.

Unfortunately, the research has only been conducted with small numbers of people, meaning that definitive conclusions can't be drawn. However, a review by the Cochrane Library in 2003 suggested that sufficient positive evidence supports reality orientation therapy to encourage people to try it.

Some criticisms

Despite the positive results that reality orientation produces, critics have suggested that repeatedly correcting a person with dementia – in terms of where she is or what day it is, for example – may actually make her worse. And taking the therapy to its extreme may mean repeatedly causing the person emotional upset. For example, a person may say she wants to go home to her husband, but is repeatedly told she can't because he died four years ago. Hearing that your spouse or parent has died when you'd forgotten about it may lead to a fresh outpouring of emotion each and every time. On a simpler level, you can easily see how being corrected about things all the time could get on your nerves and make you very irritable.

As a result of these objections to reality orientation, a few other techniques have been developed in its place:

✔ **Validation therapy:** Rather than reinforcing factual information when dealing with distress in dementia, this therapy focuses on the emotional effects of such information. Thus, for example, if the person become distressed while waiting for her father to pick her up at the care home every day, rather than saying he's long dead, the carer's response is to say he's running late and then to provide an activity to distract the person from her worries. Although this treatment can help, as yet insufficient evidence exists for it to be recommended as a treatment for all.

✔ **Specialised Early Care for Alzheimer's (SPECAL):** Penny Garner developed this treatment while looking after her mother, who had dementia. She has since set up the Contented Dementia Trust in order to share the therapy with others. SPECIAL therapy has three main rules aimed at preventing people from becoming distressed by questions their memories won't help them answer:

- Don't ask questions.

- Listen to the experts – the people with dementia – and learn from them.

- Don't contradict.

While this method no doubt reduces distress for people with dementia – and their carers – critics suggest that it disempowers people with early dementia. Not being told the truth in a particular situation means people can't be involved in decision making, something that advocates of people with dementia, such as the Alzheimer's Society, believe is very important.

Whatever the rights and wrongs of these therapies, there's no doubt that they can benefit a number of people and their carers. Recognising that everyone's different, regardless of illness and disability, means that trying some or all of these methods and seeing which, if any, are right for the person being cared for is a reasonable approach. Bespoke treatments always work better than anything 'off the peg'.

Chapter 9

Dealing with Troublesome Symptoms in Late Dementia

. . . .

In This Chapter

▶ Considering cognitive problems

▶ Managing the ups and downs of emotional symptoms

▶ Looking into functional difficulties

. . . .

*T*he later stages of each of the types of dementia can produce some of the most troublesome symptoms. In fact, they're pretty much the symptoms that come to mind when you think of a stereotypical patient suffering with dementia: wandering, disturbed nights, confusion, irritability and aggression.

By anticipating the possibility of the symptoms' arrival and looking at some of the reasons for their existence, you can take steps not only to keep them at bay but also – just as importantly – to reduce the distress experienced by the sufferer.

In this chapter I look at the issues in terms of cognitive, mood-related and functional symptoms, bearing in mind that some overlap always exists between them.

Looking at Cognitive Symptoms

Cognitive symptoms are those related to disturbances of memory and other thought processes, such as

✔ Poor short-term memory and difficulty remembering names and places

✔ Loss of judgement about money and how to adapt to the environment (wearing a coat, hat and scarf on a warm mid-summer's day)

✔ Lack of awareness of danger and the risk posed by strangers

✔ Difficulty planning tasks and problem solving

✔ Losing track of time and whereabouts

✔ Communication difficulties, including trouble following conversations and instructions and finding the right words

As dementia progresses, these symptoms often combine to make life very difficult for dementia sufferers and their carers. Here I look at some of the possible consequences of these symptoms.

Although these symptoms are common, everyone necessarily experiences them.

Wandering

This behaviour is fraught with possible danger and is the most potentially hazardous of all problems generated by dementia, because it involves the risk of

✔ Getting lost

✔ Being run over

✔ Becoming a target for muggers

✔ Developing hypothermia or becoming dehydrated as a result of wearing inappropriate clothing

Of course, none of these things may happen, and the 'wanderer' may just have a lovely stroll in the fresh air. However, I've seen plenty of carers driven to their wits' end by this behaviour as the police return their relative after a night-time sojourn to the park in his pyjamas or a jaywalking expedition along the main road.

Causes

A whopping 60 per cent of people with dementia are believed to wander. But they don't do it to get on their carer's nerves or because they're mischievous; an underlying reason for this behaviour always exists. In fact, rather than being labelled as 'wandering', this behaviour should really be seen as 'walking with purpose'. It's just that family members and carers are often in the dark about what that purpose is. Some suggested causes are

✔ **Searching for something or someone:** This may be an object the person thought he'd left somewhere and can't find, a person he desperately wants to see, or if he's in new and unfamiliar surroundings then he may simply be on the hunt for something to eat or drink or for a toilet. And he may be searching for home, often somewhere he lived in the past.

✔ **Getting away from something:** Stressful or worrying situations may prompt the person with dementia to just get up and go; maybe he finds the current environment too noisy or irritating and is trying to find some peace and quiet.

✔ **Sticking to previous routines:** Apparently, old habits die hard, and this can certainly be the case when someone goes wandering. He may set off for 'work' at a particular time or make his way to the local football stadium to support a team disbanded years ago.

✔ **Responding to memory lapses:** Someone with dementia may become stuck or side-tracked halfway through a task and set off to get the 'something' he's convinced he needs to finish off the job.

✔ **Dealing with a combination of excess energy and boredom:** Simply because someone has dementia it doesn't mean that he can't get bored or want to have a change of scenery and some exercise.

Obviously, personality differences mean this list isn't exhaustive. It does, however, cover most bases.

Strategies

Carers' stress levels can go through the roof when they're looking after someone who wanders; wandering can be a very frustrating and frightening behaviour to deal with. However, having a handle on the person's reason for wandering means that the carer can take steps to control it. Here are a few tips:

✔ **Signposting:** Make things less confusing in the house or care home by sticking labels (with words or pictures) on all the doors to say which rooms are behind them and putting up small posters with arrows directing the person with dementia to the kitchen, bathroom, dining room, lounge and so on.

✔ **Camouflaging exits:** It may sound a bit simple, but making a front door look less like a front door means it won't prove such an obvious escape route. Just hang a curtain across the back of the door or paint it the same colour as the wall. Also avoid leaving front door or car keys in sight.

✔ **Ensuring that needs are met:** Avoid the need for people with dementia to wander off to the toilet, kitchen or away from a noisy environment by anticipating their needs. Ask whether they're hungry and thirsty or need the toilet; turn down the television or music if they say they can't hear themselves think.

✔ **Offering stimulation:** Boredom is frustrating at the best of times and can be particularly so if you rely on others for your care and entertainment. Keep the person you care for occupied. If he's able, encourage him to continue with his hobbies, get him to help around the house with chores, and take him out and about to get some exercise and thereby create some natural tiredness too.

✔ **Providing easy identification:** This can best be achieved by giving people small ID cards to carry in their pockets, bags, wallets or purses. These can inform people that the holder has dementia and may need help on one side, and on the other list contact details. Also consider buying some medical ID jewellery, such as from MedicAlert (`www.medicalert.org.uk`), which not only provides identification information but also a 24-hour emergency number.

✔ **Alerting the community:** It's always useful to let neighbours and local shopkeepers know of people who are prone to wandering, so that they can keep an eye out for them and give you a call if they spot them out and about. You can also leave a small amount of money with local shopkeepers and landlords, which the person can use if they turn up there.

✔ **Avoiding leaving them home alone:** Leaving someone who can wander either indoors unsupervised or locked in the car while you nip out is asking for trouble.

✔ **Using a GPS tracking device:** Radio tracking devices are available, along with back-up support, from organisations such as Project Lifesaver (`www.projectlifesaver.org`). Mobile phone apps, such as iWander (`www.itinitek.com/iWander.html`), can also pinpoint someone who's missing.

Worst-case scenario

If someone with dementia does go missing, you need a plan for tracking him down as quickly as possible. Having notified friends and local shop owners, you'll have a ready supply of lookouts to contact for help. Developing a good knowledge of your local area is also advisable so that you're familiar with paths, parks, rivers and streams, bus stops, taxi ranks and spots where people could fall and remain out of sight.

As soon as you realise that the person you're responsible for is missing, you can afford to spend a quarter of an hour or so checking these local spots and asking neighbours, taxi drivers and shopkeepers whether they've seen him. It is also worth considering that he may have gone to see relatives or to visit an old address. After that, if you've had no luck, call the police.

Always keep a recent photo of the person with you to show to the police and others if he does go missing.

Repetitive behaviour

The problem with repetitive behaviours of any kind is that they can be, well, a little repetitive and annoying. In dementia, repetitive questions, words and behaviours are especially common, which can be very wearing for relatives and carers. However, understanding the causes of particular behaviours means you can do something to combat them.

A person with dementia may adopt a wide variety of repetitive behaviours involving both words and actions, such as

✔ Asking the same questions

✔ Telling the same familiar or personally important stories over and over

✔ Making the same sound or noise over and over again

✔ Drumming fingers, tapping feet or doing other more involved repetitive actions like packing and unpacking a bag or rearranging ornaments in a room

✔ Pacing around a room

✔ Making multiple phone calls about the same subject to the same person

Causes

Causes of particular behaviours obviously vary from person to person. Mostly, however, the behaviours are in response to an unmet need or a fear; they're not simply caused by a desire to annoy carers.

Suggested causes include

✔ **Anxiety or fear:** Confusion about what's going on can make anyone unsettled, and repetitive behaviours can be a way of communicating this unease for someone who can no longer find the right words to express it clearly. Repeated phone calls to a loved one, for example, can be an attempt to find reassurance in a situation of uncertainty.

✔ **Boredom:** Lack of stimulation can be irritating, whether you have dementia or not.

✔ **Cognitive decline:** A person may simply forget that he's already done or said something, or he may perform a task and get stuck on a certain step, which he then repeats.

✔ **Comfort or confidence in being able to talk about something familiar and important to yourself:** Specific stories from childhood or time in the services can be familiar topics.

✔ **Frustration:** A situation that isn't being resolved can lead to irritability and repetitive actions such as finger drumming while the person waits impatiently for things to be sorted.

✔ **Inability to express a need or an emotion in any other way:** A person may communicate hunger, for example, by repeatedly asking, 'What's for tea?' He may express a desire to go out by putting a coat on and taking it off again.

✔ **Pain:** Something hurts but he doesn't know why and can't say.

✔ **Side effects of medication:** If someone with dementia begins to develop repetitive behaviours that he hasn't shown before, it's always worth discussing them with his doctor.

Strategies

Any change in behaviour in someone with dementia may be a sign of a physical symptom such as pain or a side effect of medication. If such behaviour persists, ask a doctor or dementia nurse to review the situation.

If no medical issue appears to underlie the behaviour and it's simply a result of dementia itself, the following tips may help:

- ✔ **Take a deep breath.** As frustrating as these behaviours can no doubt be for you as a carer, getting cross about them can be even more unsettling and anxiety-provoking for the person you're frustrated with, and may actually make them worse. Walk away from a situation that's making you angry until you've had time to cool off. And always pick your battles. If a particular behaviour doesn't obviously have an underlying cause, try to ignore it.

- ✔ **Try to use other ways of reminding your loved one that uses less energy.** If your relative is repetitively asking how and what time he's going home then a note in his pocket that simple states 'A taxi will arrive to take you home at five' can help. Instead of running through the details repeatedly, suggest he checks his note. You want to empower your loved one to be finding things out for himself.

- ✔ **Ask whether something is disturbing the person with dementia.** Make sure you maintain eye contact to demonstrate that you're really listening to his response. Be reassuring by addressing his concerns and feelings rather than showing annoyance at his actions.

- ✔ **Explain decisions and plans for the day clearly and concisely, using visual aids if needed.** Doing so can remove uncertainty about what's happening and why, and reduce anxiety.

- ✔ **Stick to a regular routine.** If possible, establish set times for getting up and going to bed, meals and activities. Try to schedule plenty of activities to avoid boredom.

- ✔ **Redirect the person's attention.** Move him on to another activity or use music as a distraction.

- ✔ **Invest in an answerphone to screen repeated calls.** You must be available for emergencies, but need your rest too.

Sundowning

As the name suggests, people in middle to late dementia may become more confused in the late afternoon and early evening (as the sun goes down). They're invariably more lucid earlier in the day and then gradually deteriorate; the extreme confusion can last through the night and is very disturbing for both people with dementia and their carers.

Sundowning is a common problem affecting around 20 per cent of dementia sufferers.

Confusion isn't the only symptom that gets worse during sundowning; it's often accompanied by a whole set of tricky problems:

- ✔ Irritability and suspicion, with associated anger and yelling
- ✔ Disorientation
- ✔ Hallucinations
- ✔ Restlessness, pacing and consequent insomnia

If sundowning with its associated problems happens every night without fail, life can become very tiring for all concerned.

Causes

No conclusive evidence as yet supports a single identifiable cause of sundowning.

Some researchers think that sundowning may be the result of damage caused by protein plaques and tangles to nerve cells in the brain's circadian pace-maker. This part of the brain, which goes by the rather highfalutin name of *suprachiasmatic nucleus*, controls the body's sleep–wake cycles and under normal circumstances allows people to be tired and sleep when it's dark, and bright, alert and ready to face the day when it's light. In Alzheimer's disease particularly, researchers think that damage to cells in the suprachiasmatic nucleus disturbs the circadian rhythms and causes the person's brain to be confused about what's going on.

While this is a beautiful theory, for now it's mostly based on research in mice; no one's sure whether the effect is the same in humans.

Other suggested triggers for sundowning are

- ✔ Discomfort resulting from hunger or pain or a need to go to the toilet.
- ✔ Fear and anxiety generated by shadows and reduced normal sensory stimulation as daylight fades. People with dementia often manifest this fear at this time of day by saying they want to go home or find their parents.
- ✔ Less need for sleep, which is reduced to only five and a half hours as we get older.
- ✔ Noisy and disruptive surroundings, especially in care homes.

Strategies

Looking for an underlying cause can often provide an answer to how best to treat the problem, so start with a check-up by the doctor or specialist nurse when sundowning first appears. Treating this symptom with sleeping pills is inappropriate. Such medication can be dangerous for elderly people, especially those with dementia, and mainly treats the carer and not the patient.

The best treatment options are

- **Bright light therapy:** This involves the person sitting by a light box that's 30 times brighter than an ordinary bulb for between half an hour and two hours per day. Used daily, this therapy can promote better sleep, normalise day–night rhythms and improve mood and agitation.

- **Dietary modifications:** Reducing intake of foods and drinks that contain stimulants like sugar and caffeine, especially in the evenings, can promote relaxation and sleep, as can having an earlier evening meal.

- **Daytime activity:** Encouraging activity and discouraging naps during the day should make the person with dementia more naturally inclined to drop off at bedtime.

- **A restful sleeping environment:** A quiet bedroom that's neither too hot nor too cold together with a dim nightlight to reduce visual confusion caused by complete darkness encourages restful sleep.

Emotional Problems

Changes in mood top the list of common emotional problems, ranging from depression to anger and irritability. One study described in the *British Journal of Psychiatry* (Savva G.M. *et al.*, 2009) found that people with dementia experienced general apathy (50.3 per cent), depression (20.5 per cent), irritability (28.8 per cent) and agitation (9 per cent). Clearly, emotional problems can be very difficult for people with dementia and their carers to deal with.

Depression

Around one in four people are believed to suffer with depression at some time in their lives. It's not simply feeling down in the dumps or being a bit crotchety, and sufferers can't sort it out by 'pulling themselves together'. Depression is a potentially severe and disabling condition that's very common in people with dementia; around one-fifth of people with Alzheimer's disease and one-third of people with the other types of dementia are affected.

Symptoms

Psychiatry textbooks describe a set list of symptoms that when ticked off lead doctors to diagnose depression. A fair amount of overlap exists between the symptoms of depression and those of dementia, thus teasing the two apart is often quite tricky for doctors. If someone has a combination of depression and dementia, it can be a real struggle to live with.

Symptoms of depression include

- ✔ Low mood and a general sense of hopelessness
- ✔ Lack of enjoyment in life, with little to look forward to
- ✔ Poor sleep – either too much (feeling tired all the time) or too little (insomnia)
- ✔ Reduced appetite and enjoyment of food
- ✔ Poor concentration
- ✔ Suicidal thoughts and even plans in very severe cases

Poor concentration can cause people to start forgetting things or becoming muddled when carrying out normally straightforward tasks. As a result, in early dementia some people may initially be diagnosed with depression, with the other symptoms of dementia only becoming clearer with time. Similarly, new-onset depression can be mistaken for worsening dementia, hence the difficulty diagnosing depression alongside dementia, despite a well-recognised list of symptoms.

Causes

Depression is, of course, a disease in its own right, and in the same way that people with dementia can be unlucky enough to have to suffer the co-existence of other conditions such as diabetes, angina, asthma or psoriasis, they can just as easily have the misfortune of dealing with depression too.

Depression on its own can occur for a whole heap of reasons, some of which go back to childhood:

- ✔ Genetics – depression can run in some families.
- ✔ Child abuse or neglect, or even lack of love and affection from parents while growing up.
- ✔ Stressful life events such as bereavement, redundancy or divorce.
- ✔ Loneliness and isolation.
- ✔ Personality factors such as chronically poor self-esteem.

✔ Alcohol and drug misuse – although used as a self-medicated pick-me-up, unfortunately alcohol and some drugs are 'downers' and lower mood instead.

✔ Long-term illnesses – dementia, the pain of arthritis, neurological conditions like Parkinson's disease or a diagnosis of cancer can also trigger low mood and a sense of futility.

Treatment

Treatment for depression and the anxiety that often accompanies it is available from your GP, who will discuss the symptoms, try to work out what's causing them and make a treatment plan with you. Depending on the severity of symptoms, these treatments range from simple lifestyle modification and extra support at the mild end of the scale right through to input from a psychiatrist and local mental health team at the more severe end.

Lifestyle modification

Simple lifestyle interventions can produce significant improvements when someone with dementia has mild depression. Interventions include

✔ Reducing loneliness and isolation by getting the person out and about and enjoying some regular exercise

✔ Sticking to routines, which can be really important in making someone with dementia feel safe and not threatened by uncertainty

✔ Enrolling the person in clubs and day centres for a change of scenery and greater social and mental stimulation

✔ Providing ongoing reassurance that the person is an important part of the family who is loved, respected and not about to be abandoned

✔ Making time to give the person treats, be that favourite meals, trips to the cinema or theatre, or visits to see children and grandchildren

Antidepressant medication

If the depression is moderate or severe, the doctor is likely to prescribe selective serotonin reuptake inhibitors (or SSRIs, if you want to avoid tongue twisting). These pills, which come in a number of varieties, have two main actions on the brain. First, they increase levels of *serotonin* (a chemical neurotransmitter in the brain that lifts mood and reduces anxiety), and second, they increase the number of receptors for serotonin, which makes the serotonin more effective.

Natural serotonin is found in bananas. A few of my patients have suggested upping their banana intake rather than taking antidepressants. Sadly, that isn't possible, because you'd need to eat tonnes of bananas to match the effectiveness of just one pill. Tablets are definitely the best way to take this medication.

Talking therapies and dementia

I naively believed that psychotherapy has very little place in the treatment of depression or distress in people with dementia. If people with dementia can't remember previous sessions, how can they be helped to move on? However, psychotherapy can be a big help, not only for individuals in a one-to-one setting, but also for groups and carers.

Psychotherapy comes in many forms and flavours depending on the training background of the therapist or counsellor. The main types available in the UK are

✔ *Cognitive behavioural therapy (CBT)*, which deals with issues in the here and now by trying to alter unhelpful thought patterns and the behaviours people exhibit as a result of them

✔ *Psychodynamic and psychoanalytic therapies*, which are based on Sigmund Freud's theories about the role of past experiences in psychological problems in later life

✔ *Humanistic therapies*, which focus on personal growth and development

✔ *Supportive therapies*, such as counselling, which provide a safe environment in which people can discuss problems and make positive changes to their lives

Research into the use of these therapies in dementia has found that, certainly in the early stages, they can be very helpful in reducing stress by enabling people to come to terms with their diagnosis and in the treatment of the anxiety and depression that often accompany it. The therapies can also be of significant benefit to partners and carers as they deal with the feelings of sadness, grief and anxiety that many experience when a loved one receives the diagnosis.

All therapies can be accessed privately, but GPs can point you in the direction of local services funded by the NHS. Psychotherapy isn't a luxury or something that's reserved for treating the hang-ups of Hollywood types; it has a valuable place in the care of all of us, and those in need should access it as soon as possible to gain maximum benefit.

SSRIs aren't addictive and, while a few minor side effects are possible in the first week or two, they provide relief from symptoms quite quickly. SSRIs are also safe to take alongside commonly prescribed dementia medication.

Psychotherapy

Psychotherapy is the other mainstay of treatment for depression – what most people know as 'talking therapy'. It usually involves face-to-face hour-long sessions with a counsellor or therapist over a number of weeks. A number of different types of therapy are available, all of which try to enable patients to get to grips with the cause of their symptoms and offer support to get them through it (see the nearby sidebar 'Talking therapies and dementia').

Psychotherapy is available on the NHS via GPs and also privately. It's helpful for people who want to avoid taking medication, but is also useful in combination with SSRIs.

Anger and irritability

A common misconception is that everyone who develops dementia becomes aggressive, hitting out at carers and shouting and screaming at strangers. Fortunately, this simply isn't true. Dementia doesn't make the behaviour of previously passive people monstrous by default. It can, however, make people more disinhibited than usual and so more likely to react excessively to certain situations. Like the rest of us, such people are reacting to something annoying, threatening or irritating, and thus are no more likely than other people to become irritated.

Causes

Anger and irritability often result from a combination of worsening dementia making life seem more uncertain and perhaps scary, and the need to rely on others for care and support, leading to misunderstandings and confrontation. We all like things done in a certain way and when people don't accede to our wishes it can often rile us. Thus if someone who was feeding me persisted in forcing in mouthful after mouthful and didn't go more slowly when I asked him to, he'd no doubt soon see the plate flying across the room or find the next spoonful pushed back into his own face.

An ABC analysis of this sort of behaviour may reveal why it's happening and any aggravating factors, such as other people's unhelpful responses, and offer potential solutions to modify it. Address the following questions:

- ✔ What situations **A**ctivate the behaviour?
- ✔ What exactly does the **B**ehaviour involve?
- ✔ What are the **C**onsequences of the behaviour?

Strategies

The ABC analysis may identify some specific ways to help individuals with their troublesome behaviour. The following steps may also be useful in reducing or eliminating the likelihood of people with dementia becoming angry and irritable:

- ✔ Treat people with respect and dignity at all times. Ask them how they'd like you to wash and dress them, for example, and don't assume your way is the best. And also tell them what you are going to do next so that they are not startled.

- ✔ Act in an unhurried and friendly manner to avoid your actions being misinterpreted as lack of care. When in a difficult situation in public, this approach also prevents things escalating.

> ✔ Ask a nurse or GP to check the person over to make sure he isn't suffering with pain, depression, constipation, an acute infection or side effects from medication.
>
> ✔ Try to offer as much reassurance as you can in strange or difficult situations such as in large crowds or when attending medical appointments. Fear often makes the best of us lash out in anger.

You'll notice that the tips above don't include the use of medication. In the past, medication was routinely prescribed to calm down 'difficult' residents in care homes; fortunately, today that approach is the very last resort, because such drugs are potentially dangerous, and difficult behaviour always has an underlying cause that can be dealt with more effectively.

Functional Symptoms

Functional symptoms include the extremely trying problem of incontinence and the potentially life-threatening issue of falls. However, if you look for and treat their underlying causes, you can often minimise their occurrence and significance.

Incontinence

In late dementia many people suffer urinary incontinence and some even become doubly incontinent. Not only is this symptom embarrassing and uncomfortable for the sufferer, but it can also be very troublesome for carers, who may be understandably squeamish about mopping up other people's waste products and have better things to do than repeatedly filling up the washing machine.

Causes

Incontinence has four main causes:

> ✔ Direct damage to nerve pathways involved in bladder and bowel control, caused by the dementia itself.
>
> ✔ Problems with the bladder or bowel themselves, such as urinary-tract infections like cystitis, weak pelvic floor muscles following childbirth, an enlarged prostate gland in men, irritable bowel syndrome, constipation with overflow or inflammatory bowel conditions such as Crohn's disease.

✔ Inability to get to the toilet because of

- Mobility issues

- A failure to actually find it as a result of memory problems

- Not being able to communicate to a carer a need for the toilet

- Functional inability to remove clothes in time

- Side effects of medication.

Strategies

Given the possible involvement of a whole lot of other medical conditions and the side effects of prescribed drugs, the first step when someone develops incontinence is a trip to the GP to check whether any of these issues are involved. If not, and if dementia itself appears to be the cause, you can still have a few strategies up your forever rolled-up sleeves to reduce the occurrence and severity of these symptoms, including

✔ **Making going to the toilet a simple business:** Label the doors of all toilets, put up signs pointing towards them throughout the house and ensure that the route is well-illuminated at night. If someone is unsteady on his feet, raised toilet seats or hand rails in the bathroom can also help. Also avoid zips and buttons on clothing, because these can prove tricky to operate in a rush. Finally, clear the bathroom of waste baskets and potted plants to minimise opportunities for mistaken identity where finding the loo is concerned.

✔ **Keeping the person regular:** This advice comprises two aspects: first, establish a routine for taking (or at the very least politely inviting) someone to the toilet regularly to avoid accidents, and second, ensure a diet rich in fruit and vegetables to prevent constipation. Faecal incontinence can be prevented by having a set daily routine for visiting the toilet to open the bowels and avoiding stimulants like too much caffeine and spicy foods.

✔ **Using Just Can't Wait cards and Radar keys:** When you're out and about, you need to make sure you know where the toilets are and carry spare clothes or pads in case of emergencies or missed emergencies. Fortunately, two useful bits of kit are also available to make life easier:

- **Just Can't Wait card:** This costs £5 and is available from the Bladder and Bowel Foundation. It's credit card sized and states that the holder has a medical condition that means he needs to use a toilet quickly. Although the card doesn't guarantee access to a toilet, it would be a mean shopkeeper or bartender who wouldn't help.

- **Radar key:** This unlocks the 9,000 disabled toilet facilities around the country. It's available for £4.50 from Disability Rights UK, which also sells guidebooks detailing the scheme and the available facilities. You can also download a free smartphone app that provides the locations of all toilets in this scheme, together with directions to them.

✔ **Stocking up on incontinence products:** A whole range of such products is available, and you can get advice about them from your GP surgery. They include incontinence pads, rubber sheets and commodes for when getting to the bathroom has become very tricky.

Falls

Falling can become an unfortunate and potentially dangerous habit of people with dementia. In fact, experiencing falls can be one of the early signs of dementia. It certainly becomes more common as dementia progresses, with around 50 per cent of sufferers having at least one fall per year, which is twice the frequency of the general elderly population. The potential consequences of falls include fractures, head injuries and even death.

Causes

Changes in the brain caused by dementia are often the main culprit when it comes to falls. These changes can impair visuospatial judgement (affecting ability to gauge widths, distances and the height of objects and obstacles), alter a person's gait itself and reduce awareness of hazards. A person with dementia rushing to the toilet or being agitated or uncomfortable as a result of pain is thus literally an accident waiting to happen.

Other medical conditions can also increase the likelihood of falls because of unsteadiness or exaggerated confusion. Examples include Parkinson's disease, arthritis, acute infections (especially of the chest or urinary tract), poor eyesight, heart conditions (causing drops in blood pressure), diseases causing vertigo (dizziness), diabetes (particularly with frequent bouts of low blood sugar) and epilepsy.

Finally, the side effects of prescribed medication can also cause people to tumble. Heart and blood pressure pills can be responsible if someone's blood pressure drops into his boots every time he gets up, but antidepressants and tablets for epilepsy can do the same. Alcohol is another risk factor, affecting balance, vision and awareness of risks, so beware the generous nightcap.

Strategies

Falls experienced by the elderly often lead to hospital admission and potentially serious complications. My grandmother tripped over the vacuum cleaner lead in her care home, broke her hip as she fell and eventually died following complications resulting from the emergency surgery. And she's sadly not alone: more than 300,000 older people per year sustain fractures after a fall, and that number's rising. In financial terms, falls experienced by the over-65s cost the NHS in excess of £2 billion per year.

Osteoporosis and dementia

A person's risk of sustaining a fracture when he falls is dramatically increased if he has osteoporosis, more commonly known as 'thin bones'. An estimated 3 million people in the UK suffer from it. But the really bad news, according to the National Osteoporosis Society, is that one in two women and one in five men over the age of 50 suffer a fracture because of poor bone health; even more disturbingly, 1,150 people die each month as a result of hip fractures alone.

Worryingly, research indicates that osteoporosis in people with dementia is under-treated. When you consider the greater likelihood of falls in this age group, it suggests that dementia patients are at much higher risk of fractures than they need to be.

Diagnosing osteoporosis is a reasonably straightforward, two-step process: first calculate a FRAX score and then analyse the result of a DEXA scan.

FRAX is a diagnostic tool that the World Health Organization developed to predict the risk of someone sustaining a fracture resulting from osteoporosis within the next ten years. Risk factors include

✔ Bone mineral density

✔ Age

✔ Gender

✔ Clinical risk factors such as body mass index, parental history of hip fracture, use of steroids, smoking, previous fractures, consuming more than three units of alcohol per day and rheumatoid arthritis

Bone mineral density is calculated using a *DEXA* scan. If density is low and the FRAX calculation indicates a high risk of fractures, prophylactic treatment is likely to be recommended. This treatment involves the patient taking a daily tablet containing calcium and vitamin D3, which strengthen bones, and weekly or monthly bisphosphonate tablets (or an injection for those who can't tolerate the pills). Bisphosphonates work by slowing down the actions of cells that break down old bones, allowing other cells time to rebuild bones aided by the calcium and vitamin D3.

Many patients say that bisphosphonate tablets are like horse pills because they are hard to swallow, and they can actually cause the oesophagus to become inflamed, so are particularly troublesome for people who already suffer with acid reflux.

In the light of the increased risk of falls in people with dementia, chat to your GP about bone health sooner rather than later to find out whether this type of treatment to strengthen bones is advisable.

To reduce people's risk of falling and maximise their chances of avoiding serious injury if they do, take the following steps:

- ✔ Ask the GP to review the person's medication in case the current prescription makes falling more likely; possibly an alternative exits.

- ✔ Ensure a quick physical check-up occurs following a fall, not only to check for injury but also to see whether an underlying cause is present, such as dipping blood pressure, painful joints or dizzy spells. Doctors may also prescribe calcium supplements to help strengthen fragile bones (see the nearby sidebar 'Osteoporosis and dementia').

- ✔ Help sufferers maintain good muscle tone and physical fitness, where possible. Keeping them active is a start, but taking them to exercise classes specifically for older people can help even more. A referral to a physiotherapist may also be useful if arthritis is affecting gait and general mobility or if balance is an issue.

- ✔ Make the environment as risk-free as possible by removing obvious hazards and obstacles and ensuring easy access around the house. An occupational therapist can sort out modifications to people's homes, such as safety rails, slopes and bed guards, and ensure that the person has any necessary walking aids such as sticks or frames. (See Chapter 11 for more on occupational therapy services.)

- ✔ Invest in a pendant alarm, so that if someone living alone falls, he can get help as soon as possible. Such alarms do involve a small cost but offer 24-hour access to an emergency helpline and direct contact with the ambulance service.

Part III
Providing Care for Your Loved One

The top five ways to navigate a carer's challenges

- **Carry out an initial stock-take of what may lie ahead.** Although everyone's different, enough similarities exist in how dementia develops for you to gain a good idea of what's coming, even if you can't predict when. The person's finances need to be in order, benefits claimed, a will drawn up and the driving authorities informed.

- **Initiate some daily routines.** To avoid the confusion that results from not knowing what will happen from one moment or day to the next, establish a routine that takes in meal times, bath times, shopping trips, days out and so on – and stick to it.

- **Find out who can help.** No matter how capable or proud you are, you won't be able to do all the caring on your own. So chat to the person's GP or specialist nurse to find out who's who in the healthcare team and when to call on them. Also identify what support social services can offer and locate clubs and support groups for people with dementia and their carers.

- **Be open to some complementary therapies.** Although such treatments aren't as tried and tested as conventional medicines, some people do find that herbal remedies and certainly aromatherapy can help ease distressing symptoms.

- **Sort out legal issues promptly.** You'll need to help the person to write a will and choose someone to take on lasting power of attorney. Doing so while the person is still capable of making decisions for himself is clearly best. Not only will he have the satisfaction of knowing that his wishes will be complied with, but you, as the carer, will also potentially avoid future legal complications.

Find out more about the lasting power of attorney and how to set one up at www.dummies.com/extras/dementia.

In this part . . .

- ✔ Look at the challenges that inevitably face someone taking on the role of carer for a loved one with dementia.

- ✔ Get a handle on the complicated world of welfare benefits, and understand how to identify and apply for those to which you and the person with dementia are entitled.

- ✔ Acknowledge that you need to look after yourself physically and mentally to stand a chance of performing well in your caring role.

- ✔ Establish a routine that works both for you and the person you're looking after.

Chapter 10

Recognising the Challenges Ahead

*R*eceiving the news that you have dementia is a big deal. Not only does it mean that you can now make sense of the array of symptoms you've been experiencing over the previous months and possibly years, but you're also faced with the knowledge that you have a completely life-changing illness. Coupled with that knowledge is the awareness that everyone around you will be affected. Life will never be the same again for any of you.

From the carer's perspective, at the time of diagnosis the person with dementia may well be only mildly affected. She may still be working, have an active social life and be playing a full part in her family and community. At this stage, when things haven't progressed too far, she should be actively involved in making important decisions regarding jobs, finances and the legacy she'll leave behind. Don't miss this opportunity!

This chapter looks at the challenges that lie ahead if you've been recently diagnosed with dementia and what your carer may face with what appears to be an uncertain future.

Breaking the News

We expect our medical notes to remain private and confidential. Generally, we only discuss our medical histories with trusted friends and relatives. We no more want to tell our next-door neighbours that we have piles or an inverted nipple than they want to share details of their anatomical abnormalities with us. On top of this air of secrecy, some conditions are so stigmatised that no one mentions a diagnosis; HIV, mental health problems and even cancer are just a few.

Unfortunately, if you're diagnosed with dementia, you have a duty to inform certain officials, and I certainly recommend telling other people too.

Discussing the diagnosis with friends and family

The people in this group don't 'need' to be told about the diagnosis for official purposes, but letting some of them know what's going on is advisable so that they can help. Obviously, you need to do so at your own pace.

This situation is rather like the choices people make when they find out they're expecting a baby. Some women want to tell absolutely everyone as soon as they know they're pregnant; others, fearing they'll jinx things, keep the news to themselves until they've passed the three-month mark. Most women fall somewhere in between, however. They tell close friends and family the news early on, because they know they'll keep quiet and also support them if things go wrong. At three months, when the bump becomes obvious or their craving for beetroot and honey sandwiches attracts attention, they tell the world at large.

Sadly, a diagnosis of dementia isn't joyful news. Rather than celebrating a new life on its way, it heralds the final journey for that person. The premise of which people to tell and not tell is similar, however. Initially, only those who will actively help and be supportive need to know, but as things progress and the symptoms of the disease become more obvious, more people must be informed to help them understand what's going on.

No right or wrong way exists in which to tell people that you or a loved one has dementia. It's a personal choice and you must be happy with how it's done.

Telling the professionals

Your family doctor presumably already knows about your diagnosis, because she has either had the unenviable task of breaking the news to you or has received correspondence from the hospital doctor or nurse who did so. You don't have to tell any other health professionals at this stage if you don't want to. Those working at the GP surgery have access to your notes and will thus be aware of the diagnosis the next time they see you.

Others won't know, however. Letting them know at an early stage is a good idea, because they can help make sure you stay in good health and, as your condition progresses, can plan your care and anticipate difficulties as you become more mentally and physically disabled by your dementia. For this reason, consider telling your

✔ Chiropodist/podiatrist

✔ Dentist

✔ Optician

✔ Physiotherapist/osteopath/chiropractor

Other non-healthcare professionals who may appreciate knowing include

✔ Accountant

✔ Bank staff

✔ Family solicitor

✔ Financial advisor

If you have a religious faith, consider informing your religious leader as soon as possible. Hopefully, she'll help you as best she can and, with your permission, will galvanise other members of the congregation to help too as your condition deteriorates.

Informing your employer

You have no choice but to inform your employer. If you intend to keep on working for as long as you can, you have to tell your boss. Doing so is very much to your advantage, because your employer has a statutory duty to try to keep you in work by making all possible reasonable adjustments to accommodate the changes in your health. If you don't tell your employer what's wrong and how it affects you, the company won't be able to help.

Your employer will want to know

✔ Details of your diagnosis

✔ The prognosis of your particular type of dementia and how it's likely to develop over the coming months and years

✔ Your current symptoms and how they affect you

✔ The risk the job poses to your current condition, so the company can review your personal health and safety issues

✔ The advantages and disadvantages to you of staying in work

With this information, your employer may be able to offer you flexible working hours, lighter duties, equipment or computer software to help you continue to manage the work, or a different job within the same company (although this clearly may affect your income).

You may also be eligible for benefits from the government's Access to Work scheme. This scheme helps people with a disability or physical or mental health condition to stay in work by providing a grant specifically to fund practical support. How much money you're entitled to depends on your condition. You can use money from the Access to Work scheme to pay for

- Adaptations to existing equipment
- Special new equipment
- Taxi fares to work, if you can't use public transport
- A support worker or job coach to help you in your workplace
- A support service if you have a mental health condition and you're absent from work or finding it difficult to work
- Disability awareness training for your colleagues
- A communicator at a job interview
- The cost of moving your equipment if you change location or job

For more detailed information on this scheme, go to `www.gov.uk/access-to-work/overview`.

Getting Your Affairs in Order

As soon as you're diagnosed with dementia, making sure that your financial affairs are in order is a good idea. Do so as soon after the diagnosis as possible, because as the disease progresses you'll sadly be increasingly less able to manage money and financial decisions by yourself and will need help from others.

While you're still deemed to have capacity, you can make certain that the choices you make are yours and yours alone. (See Chapter 15 for more details on legal issues.) You can also appoint someone to hold *lasting power of attorney*, which means that someone you trust will oversee your finances when you're no longer able to do so.

Financial considerations

Fortunately for me, my father had the foresight to sort out writing a will and organising his finances before he became ill. When he died some years later, we didn't have to deal with any unnecessary worries alongside our grief.

In contrast, I've seen patients who've been unable to pay for their spouse's funeral or even meet household bills because the bank account wasn't in both of their names.

Financial and legal matters are dealt with in more detail in Chapters 14 and 15, but here's a quick summary of what needs to be done, because the earlier you start to think of these things, the more likely they are to be done to your satisfaction.

Bills and banking

Even when you have dementia, you still have bills to pay. In fact, the flow of brown envelopes dropping through the letterbox is seemingly endless. Given that memory and planning are the two functions of the brain most affected by dementia, it's all too easy to miss payments and risk being fined or having utilities like gas and water cut off. If you hold a joint account with your partner, this may be less of a risk if she's able to sort out ongoing finances for you. But if you have a sole bank account or your other half has memory problems too, you could be in a complete pickle.

Paying all regular and predictable bills by either direct debit or standing order is the best way to avoid this problem. You can also set up a joint bank account with someone else, perhaps the person with lasting power of attorney. Banks have simplified paying-in shops with chip-and-pin technology, but this isn't so simple if you can't remember numbers because of your dementia. Other options include

- ✔ Adding a trusted person as a signatory on accounts or allowing her to speak on your behalf to utility companies.
- ✔ A chip-and-signature card, whereby you sign for goods and services rather than entering a pin number
- ✔ A stamp of your signature, if physically signing is too difficult
- ✔ Photo ID cards

Don't withdraw lots of cash in one go. You're more likely to lose it when you're out and about in town, and having piles of notes lying around at home isn't a good idea either. And always request a receipt when you draw out cash so that you, or the person with lasting power of attorney, can keep tabs on how much you've withdrawn and where – and how much you've spent.

Benefits

Chapter 14 covers benefits in detail, but again in the days soon after diagnosis it's worth remembering that you and your future carers are likely to be eligible to apply for a variety of welfare benefits. Check out your entitlements as soon as possible, because having some extra income to help with your evolving needs will make your life more comfortable.

Financial advice

Seeing an independent financial adviser as soon as you're diagnosed with dementia is a very good idea, especially if you have assets. A financial adviser can go through your incomings and outgoings and review any savings and pensions to make sure that you're on a firm financial footing. She can also anticipate and help you plan for future changes in your circumstances, such as losing your job or moving into sheltered accommodation or a care home.

Writing a will

Writing a will is very important, because without one the government will decide how your property and assets are shared out after you die. Worse still, if you're not married and have no close relatives, the Law of Intestacy 1925 states that everything goes to the Crown if no will exists.

If you care about what happens to your estate and would like particular people or organisations to have a share of your assets, you must write a will. If you decide to make a will soon after diagnosis, you will be able to express your wishes and know that they will be followed.

The relevant government website (www.gov.uk/make-will/writing-your-will) states that you should incorporate the following instructions in your will:

✔ Whom you want to benefit

✔ Who should look after any children under 18 years of age

✔ Who will sort out your estate and carry out your wishes after your death (your executor(s))

✔ What happens if the people you want to benefit die before you

You can download a standard will from the Internet or buy one in a stationer's. However, if your will is in any way complicated, you should get legal advice. The Law Society (www.lawsociety.org.uk) suggests that you seek the help of a solicitor (I say help – obviously, you pay for the privilege) if your circumstances tick any of the following boxes:

✔ Several people may make a claim on your estate when you die, because they depend on you financially.

✔ You want to include a trust in your will (perhaps to provide for young children or a disabled person, save tax or simply protect your assets in some way after you die).

✔ Your permanent home is not in the UK or you're not a British citizen.

> ✔ You live here but you have overseas property.
>
> ✔ You own all or part of a business.

A solicitor can advise you about what to bring to an appointment, but as a guide she'll want to know about savings, stocks and shares, cars, property, businesses, insurance policies, bank and building society accounts, personal valuables and any used bank notes stuffed under the mattress.

How much a solicitor charges to draw up your will depends on the solicitor's level of expertise and the complexity of your affairs.

Driving and Mobility

Being diagnosed with dementia needn't mean an instant end to your independence. And it's certainly not good to feel that you'll be trapped at home like a prisoner. Strict legal requirements apply to when you are and aren't allowed to drive a car because you have dementia. If you or your doctor decides it's time for you to stop getting behind the wheel, don't despair: lots of other means of getting out and about are available.

DVLA regulations

You have to tell the DVLA (or the DVA in Northern Ireland) if you've been diagnosed with dementia. Failure to do so can result in a fine – currently, a hefty £1,000 – or even prosecution if you're involved in an accident.

However, telling the DVLA doesn't mean that you definitely have to stop driving, unless you yourself feel too unsafe to carry on. It does, however, trigger the organisation to find out more about your condition from you or your doctor and how it may affect your ability to continue as a safe road user. The DVLA may also ask you to take a practical driving test to assess things first hand (see the nearby sidebar 'When to give up the keys' for details).

Parking badges and bus passes

Many disabled people and their families around the UK benefit from the Blue Badge scheme, which allows them to use specially allotted car parking spaces near their destinations. The person with the disability need only be

When to give up the keys

The Alzheimer's Society (www.alzheimers.org.uk) suggests, in its 'Driving and Dementia' factsheet, that you need to think about stopping driving when

✔ You feel less confident behind the wheel or are more irritated by other drivers.

✔ You get lost, even on roads you know well.

✔ You begin to misjudge speed or distance.

✔ You find yourself straying across lanes or hitting kerbs.

✔ You become confused if, for example, road-works are taking place on a familiar route.

✔ You feel at greater risk of having an accident.

✔ Your passengers are concerned about your driving.

After many years of motoring, giving up your car and the independence it brings is hard. However, driving is a risky business, and if you're not completely capable of doing it safely, you endanger not only your life but also the lives of your passengers, pedestrians and other road users.

If in doubt, speak to your GP or specialist nurse, who can advise you further. She can also point out some of the ways in which you can be helped to stay mobile without your car.

---

a passenger in the car for it to qualify for a Blue Badge. Strict criteria govern who is and isn't eligible for a Blue Badge. Currently, people automatically qualify if they

✔ Receive the higher rate of the mobility component of the Disability Living Allowance

✔ Are registered blind

✔ Receive a War Pensioners' Mobility Supplement

According to the NHS website (www.nhs.uk), a Blue Badge may also be issued if the person

✔ Has a 'permanent and substantial' disability that makes walking very difficult or means she can't walk at all

✔ Drives regularly, has a severe disability in both arms, and is unable to operate all or some types of parking meter (or would find it very difficult to do so)

Blue Badges are thus not automatically issued to everyone with dementia – only those people who also have a physical disability or a type of dementia that causes problems with walking, particularly vascular dementia or Lewy body disease.

If driving and Blue Badges are out, another way to maintain independent mobility is to apply for a disabled person's bus pass. Issued by local authorities, such passes are known by different names throughout the UK. They're available to people who've been refused a driving licence on medical grounds, so that includes those with dementia. In some places, a companion can also apply for a pass on the grounds that she offers assistance to the disabled person while using public transport.

To find out more, contact your local council's transport department directly or search for the relevant local authority on the government website (www.gov.uk).

Taking Care of Your Health

General good health makes things easier for both people with dementia and their carers.

Dementia makes people more at risk of developing a number of physical illnesses. Some of these are disease dependent; for example, vascular dementia means a person is more at risk of heart disease and strokes. Other conditions become more likely simply because of the general debilitating effects of dementia. Potential problems include

- ✔ Constipation
- ✔ Dental issues
- ✔ Eating and swallowing difficulties and weight loss
- ✔ Thinning of the bones
- ✔ Increased risk of falls and fractures
- ✔ Incontinence of bowels and bladder
- ✔ Muscle tremors and weakness
- ✔ Kidney disease resulting from poor fluid intake
- ✔ Pneumonia and other infections because of general debility
- ✔ Skin ulcers and infections caused by poor hygiene and immobility

Experiencing the problems on this list is by no means inevitable, however, and you can try to avoid them by staying as healthy, fit and active as possible.

Alongside watching what you eat and drink and how much rest and exercise you get (see Chapter 11 for details), also using the many healthcare professionals available to monitor how well you're doing makes good sense. Let's face it, they'll only be twiddling their thumbs otherwise.

Taking the practical driving test

If you're not sure whether you're fit to carry on driving, you can take a practical driving test to see whether you're up to it. Of course, if the DVLA requests it, you have no choice but to undergo this test. You must demonstrate that you know the Highway Code and can apply it when behind the wheel of your car, and prove that you can drive safely in different road and traffic conditions. If you're referred to a mobility and driving centre by your GP or nurse then the assessment is free. If you self-refer, you'll have to pay a fee.

This test, which lasts one and a half to two hours, takes place at specific mobility centres around the UK rather than in traditional driving test centres and involves the following:

✔ Reading a number plate at a set distance to check your eyesight.

✔ Driver strength and movement will be checked, such as the pressure you're able to apply to the brake and accelerator and your reaction times from accelerator to brake.

✔ Answering two vehicle safety questions of the 'tell me, show me' variety. The 'tell me' part may involve you telling the examiner how you'd check that your fog lights are working; the 'show me' part may be demonstrating how to put air in your tyres.

✔ Driving around for about 40 minutes. For the first 30 minutes, the instructor will give you instructions and watch how you perform. You'll be asked to do hill starts, reversing, three-point turns and parking, for example. For the final 10 minutes of the test, the instructor will observe you driving independently without instructions to see how safe you are in traffic.

✔ If appropriate, an occupational therapist may use some cognitive tests relevant to driving, which will take approximately another 30 minutes.

You can take someone with you to the test to sit in the back of the car while you drive and listen to the result.

Ideally, you'll visit the following:

✔ **GP surgery:** If you have any other chronic illnesses, such as epilepsy, diabetes or high blood pressure, you should attend the surgery regularly so that the practice nurses and GPs can monitor your condition. If you're normally fit, well and on no medication but over the age of 40, you're eligible for a free NHS health check to identify risk factors for heart and kidney disease. Practice nurses are also happy to advise you about general health, diet and exercise and on how to keep your cholesterol under control.

✔ **Dentist:** Problems with your teeth and gums can make eating and drinking difficult, not to mention painful if you develop infections, mouth ulcers or abscesses. And if you don't have teeth, you need to be aware that dentures can become ill-fitting and painful too. See your dentist at least every six months for a check-up.

- ✔ **Optician:** As you get older, your eyes can fall prey to all sorts of conditions that make vision deteriorate and increase confusion and the chance of experiencing visual hallucinations. At their most simple, such conditions include short- or long-sightedness, but cataracts, glaucoma, flashes and floaters, and problems with the retina at the back of the eye are also possible. An annual visit to the optician helps pick up problems early so that they can be treated before they become too disabling.

- ✔ **Chiropodist/podiatrist:** Bad foot care puts you at risk of developing corns, in-growing toenails and infections, and suffering pain as a result. All these can also affect mobility and stop you exercising and staying fit. Paying regular trips to a chiropodist, either as a private patient or after referral on the NHS by your practice nurse or GP, allows problems to be prevented altogether or treated early.

- ✔ **Audiologist:** Your hearing levels commonly drop as you get older. The more noise the auditory nerves have had to deal with over the years – from people working in factories and on building sites or going to live gigs – the more likely they are to go on strike and make 'pardon' your most frequently uttered word. Sound conduction problems caused by something as simple as wax can also result in hearing impairment. And reduced hearing can lead to confusion – the last thing you need! If your hearing seems to be getting worse, ask your practice nurse or GP to check your ears for wax, and also get a referral to an audiologist for a hearing test.

The stronger and healthier you and your carer feel, the better able you are to cope with the challenges ahead.

Chapter 11

Making Caring Easier

*N*ot everyone is born to be a carer for someone else, particularly other adults. Yet the wedding vows we say to our spouses usually include the proclamation that we will love them in sickness and in health; therefore, when sickness such as dementia strikes, it seems only right that we step up, roll up our sleeves and get on with the job of caring. Likewise, it would be extremely unfair if as sons or daughters who were looked after by our parents as children we didn't lovingly reverse the role when those same parents are no longer able to look after themselves.

But being a carer isn't easy, and the cognitive and behavioural changes that accompany dementia can make caring for someone you love even more difficult. And that's not to mention the potential problems created by incontinence.

While at some point it may be necessary to employ professional carers, if the person with dementia is your spouse, a close friend or family member, you may still be involved in looking after him to one degree or another. This chapter provides hints and tips about how to make that role as straightforward as possible, while pointing out some of the common errors and pitfalls that can make life harder.

Being a carer isn't easy, but it doesn't have to be impossible and can actually be extremely rewarding.

Establishing Daytime Routines

Sticking to regular daily routines and schedules makes life much less confusing for the person with dementia and also allows you, as a carer, to know what you're supposed to be up to, when and on which days. In theory, a set schedule is a win–win situation all round.

Most of us feel better when our days are planned, and it can make us anxious when things go awry. I set the alarm for six thirty every workday, am in the car by seven, am at work before half past drinking a strong cup of coffee and then I get on with some paperwork before starting my morning surgery an hour later, at half past eight.

Later, I have prescriptions to sign, home visits to do and more paperwork to make an attempt to stay on top of before starting evening surgery at half past three and working until half past six or so. Then I tidy up any urgent odds and ends of paperwork before driving home. And I repeat this pattern the next day and so on.

One day a week, however, I'm on call. I still have the routine surgeries in the morning and afternoon, but can have any number of extra patients fitted into them, multiple interruptions for urgent queries from admin staff, requests to review patients' wounds from the practice nurses, possible emergency home visits, and random phone calls about patients from hospitals, ambulance crews and sometimes even the police.

During these on-call days my routine is disturbed, which is both disorientating and stressful. I often drive home from work in the evening feeling anxious that I've forgotten to do something because of the confusion caused by my haphazard workload. I really don't enjoy days like that, but experience them only once a week. And I don't have dementia.

If I had dementia and every day was as random and unplanned as my on-call day, no doubt I'd be very agitated and confused – and all for good reason.

Designing a Routine that Works

No off-the-peg, ready-to-wear daily routine exists for everyone with dementia, because no two people are exactly the same. We all have different likes, dislikes and physical needs. So my telling you to take the person out for a walk every day would be useless advice if he's in a wheelchair. Likewise, if someone hates singing and always has done, pushing him towards a music therapy session will really upset him. The plan has to be tailor-made to fit the individual.

Clearly, a daily plan has to work for you as the carer too. Thus if you need to pick up your children from school at half past three, signing the pair of you up for a session at a memory cafe at the same time is pointless.

Before working out a suitable routine for the person with dementia, consider the following:

- ✔ His previous routine

- ✔ His interests, strengths, weaknesses and physical abilities

- ✔ His 'best' times of the day, both physically and mentally

- ✔ How long necessities like washing, dressing and eating meals take

- ✔ His bedtime routine

- ✔ The timing and location of suitable clubs or events

- ✔ Your own daily needs

- ✔ Flexibility for unexpected opportunities, interruptions and visits from others

Taking these considerations into account, you can then establish a routine for each day of the week.

Review the routine after a trial period to see what works and what doesn't, which times of the week are perhaps too busy and which leave you and the person you're caring for twiddling your thumbs.

The routine will also have to be tweaked as the dementia progresses. Alterations to accommodate the person's changing needs and abilities are inevitable as time goes on. Whatever happens, however, a routine is still a good idea.

Create a simple chart detailing the events of each day and place it on the wall in an obvious place so that both of you know what's going on. Also keeping a write-on/wipe-off board to write more temporary notes and reminders can be helpful.

Simplifying Washing and Dressing

These tasks may seem simple, things we can do with our eyes closed in a matter of minutes. But to perform them quickly and appropriately requires

- ✔ Awareness that they need doing

- ✔ Ability to plan in which order to do what, from the need to take off pyjamas before putting on clean clothes, to knowing that it's best to have a wash before getting dressed rather than after in order to have more of the body available to clean

✓ Awareness of the risks of drawing a bath full of hot water

✓ Realisation that it's important to put on clean clothes and put dirty ones in the wash

✓ An appreciation of which are the appropriate clothes to wear for the weather conditions

✓ Physical dexterity and balance, which can obviously restrict a person's ability to perform these tasks on his own

Washing and dressing are also activities that can provoke embarrassment, because they're usually private and but now may involve undressing and being naked in front of someone else. They may also involve loss of self-esteem for someone who's washed and dressed himself since childhood but now needs help with such seemingly simple tasks.

And finally, it's important to remember that diving in to help, often in frustration, is not necessarily the best approach to take. People can quickly become lazy and deskilled and rapidly lose what independence they had left. So encourage the person with dementia to do as much as possible for himself, even if it takes longer.

Ensuring dignity and independence

'Do unto others as you would have them do unto you' is pretty appropriate advice for a carer. Let's face it, if the roles were reversed, we'd all have pretty strong feelings about how certain intimate tasks should and should not be performed on us. For example, if someone unceremoniously pulled your clothes off, leaving you naked, you'd probably be a little bit disgruntled. If that person then escorted you into a lukewarm shower and scrubbed you with a sponge on a stick, you'd no doubt lose the plot.

Unfortunately, I do hear of even well-meaning family members and carers washing and bathing people in this way. And, worse still, saying, 'Well, it doesn't matter because he won't remember anyway.' Actually, neuropsychological research suggests that the emotional memory of people with dementia remains intact. As a result, they can remember when they've been cruelly treated (the nearby sidebar 'Emotional memory' has the details).

Everyone deserves to be treated with dignity and respect.

Not wanting to dwell on the negative implications of the way in which you help someone you're caring for to wash and dress (and do pretty much anything for that matter), let's now consider something you can do to have a positive impact on him: encourage independence.

Emotional memory

Experiments in 1911 by Swiss neurologist Édouard Claparède provided the first inkling that even people with memory loss retain emotional memories. One of the neurologist's patients was a woman with severe amnesia. Her memory was so bad that every time Édouard met her on the ward, which could be many times during the day, he had to reintroduce himself, because she'd forgotten who he was.

One day when he shook her hand to say hello, he was holding a small, sharp tack, which pricked and hurt her. The next time she saw him, even though she couldn't remember ever having seen him before and couldn't explain why, she refused to shake his hand.

Since then many more experiments using brain-scanning techniques have discovered the different nerve pathways involved in emotional memories that are preserved in dementia, particularly Alzheimer's disease. And other research has shown that, despite significant memory loss, people with dementia retain memories of hurt, sadness and pain. They're therefore likely to behave in an agitated or frightened manner when circumstances they can remember from the past (particularly about the ways in which they've been treated by others) repeat themselves.

The flip side of this, though, is that scientists have also suggested that memories for events can be retained better by people with Alzheimer's disease if they are associated with positive emotions at the time they occur.

We all know how good it feels to be able to do things ourselves, the way we want to. It's an empowering experience, especially when we're doing things for the first time. It can also be empowering for people with dementia, who can see their previous capabilities slipping away from them, to know they can still do some things for themselves and that you still value their efforts.

It may be that you can't leave the person with dementia completely to his own devices when washing or dressing, a situation that will become increasingly obvious as the condition progresses, but by the two of you sharing tasks, he'll certainly feel he has an important part to play.

Doing it together

Here I give some tips about how to work collaboratively when helping the person with dementia with washing and dressing. And I throw in a few other bits of advice for good measure. Some of them will strike you as obvious, but others involve putting yourself in the shoes of the person and seeing things from his perspective.

Washing routines

To encourage independence and ensure that the process goes smoothly and safely

- ✔ Offer the choice of either bath or shower, and go with whichever option he prefers.

- ✔ Go shopping together and let the person choose the soap, shampoo, conditioner, bubble bath, toothpaste and other toiletries he wants.

- ✔ Be kind and not irritated when offering tips about which step comes next in the process; holding out the soap or towel at the appropriate moment can be helpful.

- ✔ Try to make ablutions a relaxing and enjoyable experience with nice fragrances and time to relax and chat, rather than a rush that suggests you have better things to do. Make it something the person looks forward to rather than dreads.

- ✔ Make sure everything you need is nearby to avoid a kerfuffle at a crucial moment; for example, towels, flannels, shampoo, a hairbrush and perhaps soothing moisturiser for afterwards.

- ✔ Always make sure the floor isn't slippery, that the water temperature is just right (for the other person, not you), that he can't get locked in the bathroom, that you're available to help without distractions and interruptions, and that bleach bottles and cleaning products aren't around to be mistaken for shower gel.

Dressing routines

We all have our favourite types, styles and colours of clothes, which all contribute to our sense of self. They don't say 'you are what you wear' for nothing. Thus being told what to wear can stifle independence. To encourage people with dementia to dress themselves:

- ✔ Make sure the room is warm and privacy respected as far as practicable. Close the curtains, and if the person needs help, try to provide a carer of the same gender.

- ✔ Lay out clothes in the order in which they should be put on, so that trousers don't precede pants, and shoes aren't put on before socks.

- ✔ Choose clothing with simple fasteners – Velcro straps rather than laces, zips not buttons.

- ✔ Lay out clothes so that they're easy to get into and out of; doing so makes the job simpler and much less likely to cause anger, frustration or embarrassment.

✔ Put out a choice of clothes to allow the person to choose what he wears. Don't get irritated if he puts patterns or colours together that you don't think work or don't think are appropriate.

✔ Change what's in the wardrobe according to the seasons, so that the person's attire is appropriate.

✔ Go shopping together so that his wardrobe is updated and fashionable and he has new items to choose from. Allow him to choose the shops he wants to go in and the clothes he wants to buy. Help him in the changing room or buy the same item in a couple of sizes to take home and try on; you can return unsuitable items later.

✔ Allow time for dressing so that the process isn't a stressful rush for either of you.

Washing and dressing are important elements of helping people to feel calm, relaxed and good about themselves. Don't turn these activities into a chore or, worse still, a battle. These experiences can set the tone for the day. It can be a lengthy process, though, so patience is needed.

Handy gadgets

As time goes on, both bathing and dressing can become distinctly tricky procedures for someone with dementia. As a result, they can be tricky procedures for carers to facilitate too.

Thankfully, a variety of gadgets designed to help with these activities is available online and in shops specialising in disability aids. The person's GP can also refer you to an occupational therapist, who will undertake an assessment, offer advice on suitable aids and actually supply some of them.

Washing aids

Loads of aids are available to help with bathing and showering, such as

✔ Inflatable bath pillows, to allow someone to lie back comfortably as he soaks

✔ Anti-slip bath mats to prevent falls getting into and out of the bath

✔ Bath seats to allow those who can't get right in and sit on the bottom to bathe, albeit in shallower water

✔ Tap turners for people with weak hands or problems with co-ordination

✔ Steps to help people get into and out of the bath without having to step over the side in one go

✔ A walk-in shower or wet room can be really useful for those with compromised mobility or those who needed assistance

✔ Bath and toilet grab rails

✔ Shower mats

✔ Shower seats

✔ Long-handled back brushes

✔ Mobile shower chairs

Dressing aids

These aids are designed to help with fiddly tasks while dressing, and thereby increase independence:

✔ Non-tie shoelaces, which are made of elastic, don't need tying or untying, and aren't long enough to trip over

✔ Sock and stocking aids, which have long cotton tapes attached, allowing footwear to be pulled up easily

✔ Button hooks, which are pretty self-explanatory and allow fiddly buttons to be pulled through button holes easily

✔ Long-handled shoehorns, which prevent the need to bend when putting shoes on

Managing Diet and Eating Difficulties

Food isn't just a basic human necessity; it also provides opportunities for enjoyment and socialising. In fact, the act of preparing food can also be a source of stimulating physical and mental activity.

Thus, although nutrition and energy are essential for human survival, regardless of whether you have dementia, preparing meals and sharing them with others can be just as important in terms of their therapeutic value. And while we may not all be Jamie Oliver, amateur cheffing can still be fun.

Getting five a day

However much we may enjoy a hearty English breakfast, tea and cake, or fish and chips, they're not enough to sustain us. We need a mixed and balanced diet of protein, carbohydrate, fats, sugars, vitamins and minerals, fibre and water. A healthy diet is particularly important for people with dementia, to help them keep their strength up and remain fit for as long as possible, and thereby maintain their independence. Poor nourishment adds to the risk of falls and of succumbing to all kinds of infections and other illnesses.

A vital part of a balanced diet is the infamous five portions of fruit and vegetables per day. These foods not only provide a rich source of vitamins, minerals and disease-preventing antioxidants, but also contain plenty of fibre to produce firm stools and keep the bowels moving, thus reducing the risk of incontinence.

Here's a quick run-down of the kinds of foods that can be used to add up to the magic number five. How much is needed of each varies and nowadays is often printed on the side of the packet:

- Fresh fruit and vegetables – a medium-sized piece of each counts as one portion; for melons and grapefruits, a quarter suffices
- Beans and pulses, which count as one portion no matter how many different types you eat
- Frozen fruit and vegetables
- Tinned fruit and vegetables
- Dried fruit
- Vegetables in microwave ready meals (although beware the unhealthy levels of fat and sugar in most such meals)
- Vegetable soups
- Fruit juices and smoothies

A very wide variety of fruit and veg is available and can suit most tastes and budgets. Providing these famous five portions, in whatever form, is what's important.

Encouraging a balanced diet

Of course, fruit and veg are only part of what forms a truly balanced diet. Alongside these foods we all need a selection of other goodies:

- **Proteins:** These help build strength by maintaining muscle bulk, and are found in milk, yoghurt, eggs, seafood, nuts, meat and soya products, meaning that both vegetarians and meat eaters can get their fair share.
- **Carbohydrates:** This group of foods helps provide energy. Rice, pasta, couscous, potatoes, bread and breakfast cereals are all good sources.

✔ **Fats:** While a low-fat diet is generally thought to be healthy, we do need some fats to keep our bodies ticking over. Healthy sources of fat are oily fish, low-fat milk and cheeses, olive oil and margarine.

✔ **Fibre:** This is the stuff that keeps our bowels regular. Fibre can be particularly important for people with dementia, because relative inactivity and some dementia medications can predispose them to constipation. Foods that are high in fibre include breakfast cereals, brown rice, potatoes with their jackets on, fruit, veg, beans and lentils.

✔ **Calcium:** This mineral is found in milk, cheese and most other dairy products. It's important for keeping bones strong and reducing the risk of breaks from falls.

Including some of each of these food groups in the diet of someone with dementia is vital if he's to remain as healthy as possible for as long as possible. And going to the supermarket or local shops together to choose food can be another part of the weekly activity plan.

If the person with dementia lives alone or is left alone for long periods during the day, he may either forget to eat or simply forget where the food is. Placing a bowl of fruit and snacks in easy sight and reach can be helpful. The visual prompt helps him know when to eat or question whether he's hungry.

Getting fluids in

Keeping track of fluid intake is important to ensure your loved one doesn't get dehydrated. Dehydration can cause confusion in its own right or make urine infections more likely, which can again cause confusion. Leaving a jug of water or juice in near reach or plain sight will give someone a visual reminder to have a drink. And other ways of increasing fluid intake without pushing drinks are to have soup, ice lollies, ice cream, jelly and blancmange. Anything with a high fluid content will help.

Never too many cooks: Getting the person involved

Cooking can easily be a joint effort, involving the person with dementia throughout the process to keep him both occupied and mentally stimulated. You can plan for a cooking session every day or as a special event once or twice a week.

A vast array of cookbooks and downloadable recipes is available for you to choose from. Of course, you may have your own favourites, but trying different things makes mealtimes less boring, and following recipes helps people with dementia maintain confidence in their abilities and builds their self-esteem. Maybe cooking has always been their thing, and the fact that they're still able to prepare their signature dishes will provide a tremendous boost in confidence.

Given that dementia affects memory and planning, to avoid frustration, breaking down cooking tasks into small, manageable chunks is best. You also need to make sure that people with dementia are supervised if they're using potentially hazardous pieces of kitchen equipment such as sharp knives or boiling water in a saucepan. Metal and microwave ovens also don't go well together.

While you may have to supervise and keep an eye on timing, you can nonetheless allocate individual tasks in the order in which they have to be carried out:

- Washing and peeling vegetables
- Chopping and boiling vegetables
- Buttering bread ready to make sandwiches
- Making a cuppa for afternoon tea
- Washing or drying up afterwards (or unloading the dishwasher)

Meals on wheels

For those without family nearby, or who live alone and aren't safe or able to prepare their own meals, healthy, balanced foods can be delivered directly to them. The meals on wheels service is provided by most local councils around the country (go to www.gov.uk/meals-home to find your nearest provider) and also by private companies.

Local authorities

Arrangements no doubt vary around the country, but as a guide to the sort of service provided, here's the way it works for my patients in Bristol:

- Anyone can apply to be part of the scheme, without the need for a referral from his GP or social services.
- You can set up the service for yourself, a relative, friend or neighbour.
- Hot meals are delivered anytime between 11 a.m. and 3 p.m. They're ready to eat straightaway and can be provided seven days a week if needed.
- A sandwich or cold salad tea can also be delivered at the same time ready for later on.

✔ A wide choice of foods is available, catering for all tastes (from Indian and Chinese dishes to traditional meat and two veg) and special dietary requirements.

✔ The person delivering the meals helps clients to get started with their food, if needed, by fetching cutlery, opening lids and so on. The delivery person also checks that clients are okay, and will call a relative or doctor if he has concerns.

This great service, run by volunteers, provides not only good food but also reassurance that the person with dementia is checked on every day. You can contact your local council or check its website for details of the services near you. Meals on wheels charges vary across the country from council to council, but are in the region of £5 per day for a hot meal with a pudding.

Private companies

Home food delivery services have sprung up around the country and can be found on the Internet or in local telephone directories. Like council providers, many provide daily hot meals, but some companies also deliver frozen meals that can be reheated when needed. This service provides the flexibility of being able to have meals out or with family without wasting a hot delivered meal or getting in a pickle about cancelling a delivery. It also means that people have more choice about what they fancy eating on a particular day. Of course, this service is only suitable for people who are still fully able to operate a microwave or conventional oven safely and able to check that food is heated through thoroughly before eating it.

An extensive array of foods is available, and all dietary and religious needs are catered for. The cost of individual meals varies, but delivery is often free. Check company websites for details. Individual meals are useful because families can easily check on whether they are being eaten regularly by how many are left at the end of the week.

Helping when eating becomes tough

You can have the most appetising-looking meals created by the finest chefs and delivered directly to your plate, but if the mechanics of physically eating them start to let you down then getting any nourishment from the food, let alone enjoying the tastes and flavours, can be very difficult. Sadly, as dementia progresses, not only do people go off their food and lose their appetite, but they also begin to struggle to eat and swallow. The physical dexterity necessary for wielding cutlery also begins to fail, meaning the whole process becomes a struggle.

Stimulating an appetite

Bland, boring food is a turn-off for all of us, hence the age-old jokes and moans about school dinners and hospital food. Nothing's worse than being served up either the same food day after day or food that you don't like.

Try these ideas for keeping people with dementia interested in their food:

✔ Encourage them to eat little and often.

✔ Give them a choice and involve them in preparation if possible.

✔ Use strong flavours and good seasoning.

✔ Offer sweet, tasty desserts.

✔ Provide softer foods if chewing is a problem.

✔ Try finger foods, milkshakes and smoothies, which can be easier to get down while still providing plenty of nutrients.

✔ Turn off the TV and cut down on other distractions and noise, so that they can focus on what they're eating.

✔ Make mealtimes relaxed and sociable occasions rather than battle-grounds for disputes about nourishment.

✔ Ensure that no obvious physical obstructions to enjoying food exist, such as ill-fitting dentures or problems with teeth, by taking them for regular dental check-ups.

✔ Check that they're wearing their glasses, if they have them; they may not fancy eating simply because they can't see what you're offering.

Dealing with problems getting hand to mouth

If co-ordination fails as dementia progresses, getting started with a meal, let alone finishing it, can be difficult and embarrassing. The fear of tipping things up, spilling drinks, dropping food on the table or floor, and having a face covered in sauce like a toddler with an ice cream can be very stressful for an adult intent on maintaining dignity.

Being aware of co-ordination difficulties is important, because they can stifle the person's desire to eat, for fear of looking foolish. Thankfully, this problem can be worked around very easily:

✔ Chop food up to make it easier to get onto a fork and into the mouth.

✔ Encourage the person to use a spoon if a knife and fork is proving too fiddly.

✔ Provide finger foods such as cocktail sausages and chopped raw vege-tables for lunch and snacks rather than 'doorstep' sandwiches or soup.

✔ Invest in specially designed cutlery, cups and tableware aimed at help-ing people who have difficulty gripping or difficulty with co-ordination to maintain independence; you can buy cutlery with easy-grip handles or angled heads, non-spill cups, partitioned bowls and plates, angled bowls and plate surrounds to make scooping easier.

Aiding with chewing and swallowing

Even when food has been successfully brought from the plate to the person's mouth, the eating process is still not complete and it's a long way from the mouth to the stomach without some help. Sadly, people with dementia may forget to chew or may experience physical difficulty chewing and swallowing.

As my grandmother's dementia advanced, mealtimes became long, pro-tracted affairs. She'd still be halfway through the first course while we, had we not waited, could have been scraping the last scoops of dessert from our bowls. She was a talker too, which didn't help. Even when we cut up her food, she forgot to chew and would hold food in her mouth for minutes at a time before responding to reminders to get chomping. She did benefit, how-ever, from being given smaller portions and softer foods – and from being reminded to quit nattering and get on with eating!

A speech and language therapist can provide advice on eating and swallowing difficulties. If the preceding tips don't help, ask the person's GP for a referral.

Finally, if things reach the stage where independent feeding is neither pos-sible nor safe, you can feed the person yourself and also ask the GP to supply nutrient-rich drinks, shakes and mousses to ensure the person makes up the deficit resulting from smaller meals.

Getting Out and About

Boredom's a killer. Nothing's worse than having to spend day after day star-ing at the same four walls with no hope of change in environment or circum-stances. It's isolating, lonely and depressing. But getting fresh air, a change of scenery and some gentle exercise is invigorating and stimulating, and pro-vides a boost to people's moods and emotions. This applies whether you're 9 or 90, with or without dementia. If you do have dementia, however, getting out and about can be a vital way of staying fit and mentally and physically active for longer.

Providing fresh air and exercise

Everyone should try to get at least half an hour's exercise five days a week in order to stay fit and healthy. Exercise keeps the heart ticking over nicely, strengthens bones, helps prevent insomnia and keeps the body supple. And evidence suggests that exercise can reduce the rate of cognitive decline in people with dementia too.

As we get older, exercising can become more difficult as osteoarthritis makes joints stiff and painful, balance deserts us and energy levels aren't what they used to be. These difficulties can be exacerbated by certain types of dementia, such as Lewy body disease and vascular dementia, whereby mobility can be affected by disease processes in the brain.

Not everyone with dementia is old or physically incapacitated, however, and exercise and activity outside the home or in the garden can help maintain mobility and independence for longer. Getting out and about also increases opportunities to meet new people and makes life generally more interesting.

If you're worried that the person you're caring for is a bit out of shape or has other medical conditions that may be adversely affected by exercise, by all means ask his GP or practice nurse to check him over and advise on what he should and shouldn't do. But given that exercise helps most conditions, the person is more than likely to be given the thumbs-up.

Exercise need not mean training for marathons or squeezing into Lycra and heading to the gym. The following activities are fantastic ways for people with dementia to keep fit:

✔ Gardening

✔ Swimming

✔ Tai chi

✔ Pilates

✔ Walking

✔ Bowls and skittles

✔ Dancing

If the person is up to it physically, the only limitation to what's possible is your (and his) imagination. Exercise needn't stop in the later stages of dementia, although it will obviously have to be adapted. People can still be encouraged to go for a walk, potter around the garden or simply do stretches and upper-body exercises if their legs have gone on strike. People who are wheelchair-bound also benefit immensely from getting outside regularly for fresh air and a change of scenery.

Helping people become ladies (and gents) that lunch

Socialising with others is another great way to try to prevent boredom and cognitive decline, and for those to whom exercise is an anathema, meeting others at a club or coffee shop can be an excuse to get them out of the house and walking about too.

Many age-related and dementia charities run cafes particularly set up so that people with dementia and their carers can enjoy a tea or coffee and take part in stimulating activities such as quizzes, reminiscence work and music therapy. Go to www.memorycafes.org.uk to access the list of these cafes throughout the UK.

You can also organise informal social events, factoring trips for lunch and coffee into the person's weekly schedule, and getting friends and family around for games evenings in the person's home. Life need not be sedentary or boring!

Staying on Top of Health Care Issues

In the UK, we're blessed with an amazing NHS that's free at the point of need to everyone, no matter how much or little they earn or the list of medical conditions afflicting them. This isn't the case everywhere in the world, and people with dementia in other countries who can't afford to pay for their health care can become unnecessarily disabled as a result.

Making good and sensible use of what we have is thus important. People with dementia obviously need help with and advice about whichever disease is producing their symptoms. But they may also have other medical conditions such as diabetes, high blood pressure, asthma, thyroid disease, arthritis and menopausal symptoms that also need keeping an eye on. The list is endless because old age also throws up lots of new problems that a doctor needs to cast an eye over, such as cataracts, falls, Parkinson's disease, heart attacks and strokes.

People with chronic diseases (diabetes, high blood pressure and so on) are invited to attend monitoring clinics run by practice nurses at their GP surgery. Keeping these appointments is vital.

Visiting doctors, dentists, podiatrists and opticians

Looking after the person's teeth, feet and eyes is important. Make sure they're checked at least annually, if not six-monthly. Prevention is always better than cure.

If you're unable to get the person you care for to an appointment under your own steam or safely on public transport, speak with your GP surgery; it may be able to arrange either a home visit or community transport.

Bear in mind that people with dementia may feel anxious about visiting the dentist or being in an unknown, potentially busy, environment. Behavioural problems and agitation may result. Try to keep stress levels to a minimum by

- Attending appointments with the person with dementia to offer support and give him confidence

- Trying to attend the same clinics and see the same clinicians each time, so that the person with dementia gets used to the surroundings and personnel

- Letting the professional know that the person you are with has dementia, and giving him useful tips for minimising the potential stress of the situation for all concerned

- Taking along a list of points you want to cover with the clinician, drawn up with the person with dementia if possible

- Allowing the person with dementia to talk for himself when possible, and not irritating him by talking over him

- Not covering too much in one go and making the experience exhausting

Don't let a previously stressful visit or the person's declining dementia put you off taking him to appointments again. His physical health and eyesight are vital to him.

Coping with pills and medicines

Prescription medicines often have ridiculous names that make them hard to pronounce and remember, even for carers, let alone people with dementia. Pills for different conditions can also have extremely similar names, which can lead to confusion. Penicillin, for example, has a very close namesake – penicillamine – that's no help at all in treating infections, because it's designed to modify the symptoms of rheumatoid arthritis. And if that's not enough, drugs often go by both their generic and brand names. The capsule to treat the symptoms of reflux and heartburn can thus be known by its brand name – Losec – or its generic name – omeprazole. For all these reasons, mixing up pills is very easily done.

A person on multiple drugs for lots of different conditions could be made very ill as a result of confusing different medicines. Mixing up medications also involves the risk of under- or overdosing.

Checking what's what with the doctor

The person's GP (and sometimes the GP's clinical pharmacist) will be very happy to sit down and take you through each medicine the person you're caring for is taking and what it's treating. Try to arrange such a meeting as early as possible so that you have a clear understanding of what's going on right from the start and can then explain the situation to the person you're caring for, and repeat it as necessary each time he asks. Knowing the purpose of each medication also means you can stress the importance of taking each one and when it should be taken.

A dangerous method

Safe management of medicines is crucial to medical practice, but it can become a little haphazard in people when they begin to develop cognitive impairment. As a medical student I encountered a patient with a very idiosyncratic – and dangerous – method of deciding which medicines to take.

Tom was in his 90s and lived alone with only his dog Bess for company. He'd seen the GP because he was experiencing palpitations, but had since become a bit of a medical mystery because no matter what his doctor tried or how many times he thought he'd cracked it, Tom said he was no better.

Finally, the GP made a home visit and asked Tom to demonstrate his symptoms in his own environment. And enlightenment dawned. On the kitchen dresser was a stack of pills – as prescribed by the GP.

'Hey, Tom,' the doctor said, 'what's with all the unopened pill boxes then?'

'Ah,' said Tom, 'well, it's like this, Doctor. When you give me a new packet of pills, I always bring them back and give one to old Bess here. And if she doesn't like them, there's no way I'm going to take them meself.'

Using dosette boxes and blister packs

Ask the pharmacist to dispense the person's medication into either a dosette box or blister pack. Each method involves the pills being set out in an easy-to-follow pattern, with all tablets to be taken at a particular time of day grouped together in a blister or small tray, one for each day of the week. Prescriptions can also be delivered as weekly packs, which means that clinical staff and carers can also monitor whether all the pills are being taken. The limited supply in the person's home each week also prevents accidental overdose.

Dosette boxes and blister packs are great ways to ensure peace of mind for everyone involved in a person's care. They also encourage independence, because the person can keep administering his own medicines for as long as he's able.

Automatic pill dispensers provide another way to ensure medication is taken safely. These dispensers have the added advantage of an alarm to remind the person when to take his tablets. And having the pills safely locked in the dispenser until the allotted time minimises the chances of overdose. These dispensers can be bought online, with prices ranging from around £40 to £90. They have to be filled by family or carers.

Chapter 12

Coping with Caring

• •

In This Chapter

▶ Taking a long, hard look at the challenges facing carers

▶ Making sure you take good care of yourself and don't get burnt out

▶ Creating time for yourself

▶ Ensuring your finances add up

• •

*B*eing a carer isn't an easy job, especially if you also have a paid job, a family, friends, a social life, your own health concerns and so on. And while caring for a member of your family when her dementia renders her no longer independent can be very worthwhile and rewarding, it can also be physically, mentally and emotionally exhausting.

The caring role also comes with many uncertainties. You may wonder whether you're doing it right or whether you're missing out on available practical help and financial support. Acting as a carer is unpaid and stressful, but help is out there to make sure that you don't end up feeling overwhelmed and unable to cope.

This chapter covers not only the challenges you might expect to encounter, but also the symptoms to look out for if stress is effecting you. There are tips on how to look after yourself both physically and mentally, and advice about whom to turn to for help if you still find yourself struggling. And finally, a reminder that you are not super-human and you can only do your best.

Considering the Challenges

When my grandmother first developed dementia, my mum (her daughter) helped care for her. It wasn't an easy task. As my grandmother became less independent, my mum needed to do more for her around her flat to keep it clean and tidy in the way she knew my grandmother would like it. As Hilda became more forgetful and anxious, the frequency of phone calls increased, my grandmother asking the same questions again and again, day after day and night after night.

My grandmother become more frightened about what was happening to her, and her personality simultaneously changed: she became increasingly aggressive. My mum bore the brunt of it, often being shouted at in shops when my grandmother became muddled and confused, and once even being shoved into a wall as they walked down the street. Fortunately, my mum loved her mother dearly and was only too happy to reciprocate the care she'd received while she was growing up.

But the job was a difficult one and it kept getting harder, not least because the goalposts constantly moved. Just as my mum felt that she'd got the hang of dealing with her mother's behaviour, either the behaviour would change or my grandmother would respond differently to my mother's attempts to help. As the role became increasingly challenging, my mum began to find her mother annoying and resented having to get a bus across town to see her a couple of times a week only to be shouted at when she arrived – and then felt extremely guilty as a result.

Ultimately, my grandmother had to go into a residential care home, and my poor mum felt guilty and stressed about taking that decision too.

The challenges involved in being a carer for someone with dementia are many, varied and ever-changing as time goes on. And millions of people are facing these challenges around the clock, every single day.

Caring and stress

We become stressed in any situation where we feel we have little control over what's going on. And while some stress is thought to be good for us, prolonged and persistently high levels of stress can be bad for our health. Adrenaline, the fight or flight hormone, is responsible for creating this sensation. When we're stressed and feel under threat, the adrenal glands release more adrenalin into the blood stream to prepare our bodies to either fight it out or flee.

And while a regular shot of adrenaline was useful for early humans millions of years ago who regularly wanted to steal food or land from a neighbouring tribe or avoid a marauding woolly mammoth, it's not so helpful when you're helping a person with dementia get dressed, changing her soiled sheets for the tenth time in a day or finding her when she's gone wandering.

Effects of stress

In the short term, excessive adrenaline produces the symptoms we're all familiar with in the run-up to exams or a job interview: a sick feeling, a frequent urge to pass urine or go to the toilet to empty loose bowels, butterflies in the stomach, a racing pulse, a tight throat and inability to catch the breath.

In highly stressful situations such as caring high levels of adrenaline and its close compatriot, the hormone noradrenaline, can produce a range of unwanted physical and emotional symptoms:

- ✔ **Physical symptoms:** These include tension headaches that radiate up from the back of the neck and make the skull feel as though it's in a vice; heart palpitations; nausea; daily bowel upset, ranging from chronic constipation to abdominal pains and diarrhoea; and widespread bodily aches and pains that aren't the result of either injury or overexertion. Over the long term, blood pressure may rise, leading to an increased risk of heart attack and stroke. It's not uncommon for people experiencing unrelenting stress-related physical symptoms to start to believe they're actually seriously ill, possibly with cancer. I frequently encounter such patients seeking reassurance.

- ✔ **Emotional symptoms:** Long-term stress can play havoc with someone's mental health. Depression and anxiety are common and can lead to a whole range of other emotional responses, such as anger, irritability, sleep problems (insomnia or excessive tiredness), changes in appetite (going off food altogether and losing weight, or comfort eating and piling on the pounds), loss of interest in life (hobbies, socialising, reading, television), poor concentration for even the simplest tasks, reduced sex drive and even suicidal thoughts.

  Depression and anxiety can also lead to alcohol abuse and increased cigarette consumption. And stress and anxiety are the commonest reasons for work absenteeism in the UK.

Types of stress experienced by carers

Research has shown that the stress experienced by carers differs according to the type of dementia the person they're caring for is suffering from and the particular symptoms she's exhibiting. According to a study published in the *European Journal of Geriatric Psychiatry* in 2012, carers report the following:

- ✔ Looking after people with Lewy body disease and fronto-temporal dementia is more stressful than caring for people with Alzheimer's disease or vascular dementia.

- ✔ Psychiatric symptoms such as hallucinations, depression, anxiety and apathy in the person with dementia are a particular cause of stress.

- ✔ Fluctuations in the cared-for person's cognitive symptoms (and therefore unpredictability) are more stressful than a steady deterioration in memory and ability to plan.

- ✔ The person with dementia's age and gender and the degree of impairment in relation to carrying out activities of daily living and mobility are less likely predictors of carer stress than the factors I just listed.

Dealing with guilt

Many carers feel a sense of guilt when they're looking after loved ones with dementia. This feeling can arise for a variety of reasons, but can actually be dealt with when it's acknowledged.

We're all different, and depending on our personalities we feel guilty about some thoughts, feelings and failures and not about others. Perfectionists probably feel guilty about anything that falls below the tough standards they set themselves, while those with a more relaxed attitude probably cope better when things don't go well. Caring is a tough role whatever your personality, but particularly so if you're looking after the person with dementia 24 hours a day.

Carers feel guilty for a whole range of reasons, including

- ✔ **Comparison with other carers:** Evolution has made us a competitive species. From school and even the nursery onwards, we're encouraged to compare ourselves with others. Doing so as carers isn't helpful, though. Other people may appear to be doing a 'better' job, but that doesn't mean they actually are. They're likely to be experiencing their own struggles, doubts and guilty feelings.

- ✔ **Negative feelings towards the person being cared for:** People with dementia can be aggressive, demanding – and dirty. Caring for someone who smells, is wearing dirty clothing, looks grubby and – worst of all – is incontinent, sometimes doubly so, is very difficult. Carers may feel a sense of disgust, swiftly followed by guilt. Couple that with challenging or embarrassing behaviour, and the carer may find it difficult to like, let alone love, the person they're caring for.

- ✔ **Emotional baggage from the past:** Not all carers share a rosy history with the person they're caring for. Possibly, they feel guilty because they didn't pick up on the person's early symptoms quickly enough and were impatient and cross with her as a result. Maybe the carer treated the person with dementia as if she was daft, muddled and intentionally annoying rather than unwell.

  Even further back, maybe the carer has always had a troubled relationship with the person with dementia. Maybe the person was a poor, neglectful or abusive parent. Seeing that person become helpless and vulnerable can stir up all sorts of emotions, particularly about the carer's feelings towards her.

- ✔ **Feelings of failure when the carer can't manage alone:** Accepting help from others can be difficult, and people often feel guilty when they can no longer cope alone and have to call in the professionals. This guilt is invariably magnified if the person with dementia ends up in a care home.

Sometimes the guilt arises from carers' personal beliefs that they should do more, but it can bubble up because of pride and the notion that others will think badly of them.

✔ **Feeling trapped:** Trying to fit caring on top of a job, socialising, family time, a sex life and so on can be extremely stressful. Caring can understandably engender feelings of resentment and entrapment, followed by guilt.

✔ **Needing time out:** I know of carers who desperately need a break but feel so guilty about leaving the person with dementia on her own or with someone else even for an evening that they don't take any time to recharge their own batteries. Taking time for themselves can make carers feel so bad that they push themselves to the point of exhaustion – benefiting no one.

If you recognise any of these guilty feelings, you first need to acknowledge that they're totally normal, and not just in relation to caring but in pretty much all aspects of life and in many relationships. Second, rather than bottling them up, you need to offload those feelings by sharing them with others. Consider talking to a good friend, a sibling, other carers (who'll inevitably feel just like you!), a GP, a specialist nurse, your religious leader or a counsellor. Finally, work out ways to create some time for yourself. Doing so isn't selfish and you're not letting down the person you're looking after. In fact, recharging your batteries means you'll be better able to care for the person afterwards than if you'd soldiered on in a state of exhaustion, your guilty feelings intact.

Looking After Yourself

Every time you fly, you're given the same safety talk from the cabin crew as the aircraft begins to taxi towards take-off. And if you can hear what they're saying above the chatter of disinterested fellow travellers, you know they not only tell you how to fasten, adjust and release your seatbelt, point out the route to the plane's exits and show you the position to adopt if you hear the words 'brace, brace' (which, surprisingly, isn't on your knees in fervent prayer), but also instruct you on what to do if oxygen masks drop from the panel above.

Parents are told to put on their own oxygen masks before attempting to do so for their children. At first this instruction seems rather heartless and selfish – in a crisis, shouldn't children come first? However, it actually makes good sense. If a parent attended to her child first and then passed out because she couldn't get her own mask on in time, she'd no longer be able to take care of that child, and obviously the child can't take care of her. As soon as she has adequate oxygen, however, the adult has time to sort out and protect her child.

The same logic applies to being a carer for someone with dementia. If you don't look after yourself properly, how can you expect to have the mental and physical strength and energy to look after your more vulnerable relative?

Seeking professional support

Prevention is always better than cure, and as a doctor I'd rather advise patients about how to stay fit and healthy before they head off on their travels than have to resuscitate them on their return because they didn't take malaria pills or get vaccinated and now have a potentially life-threatening mosquito-borne illness, rampant diarrhoea and the after-effects of altitude sickness. These things are preventable with the correct physical preparation, travel jabs and pills.

Likewise, I'm always happy to chat to someone who's about to become a full-time carer to offer advice about what to expect and the physical and mental challenges ahead. And the nurses at the surgery will gladly give such people a physical MOT. Being a carer is rather like competing in an endurance sport: people wouldn't head off to run a marathon or climb a mountain without knowing they were physically up to the job and had prepared in advance.

Staying healthy

Don't think that asking for a check-up is wasting the nurse's or doctor's time. They're happy to have the opportunity to dish out the following advice:

- ✔ **Eat a healthy, balanced diet.** Ensure you get five portions of fruit and veg and plenty of water every day, and stop what you're doing and actually sit down to eat; also try to keep off the fags and booze.

- ✔ **Get some exercise.** Just a short walk around the block every day suffices to keep you in shape and raise the endorphin level in your brain to boost your feeling of wellbeing.

- ✔ **Have a good night's sleep.** You need your rest if you're to keep going day after day, so try not to wait until the person you're caring for goes to bed before you start doing chores. Doing jobs like washing and cleaning together not only gives the person with dementia a sense of purpose and some exercise, but it also allows you to have some 'down time' in the evening and to get to bed at a reasonable hour.

- ✔ **Take care of your back.** If you have to help the person with transfers into and out of bed, on and off the toilet and out of chairs, you need to be very careful with your back. While GPs can offer advice about back care, also seeing a physiotherapist is probably worthwhile. Not only can physiotherapists check out your spine in more detail and treat existing problems, but they can also show you the best way to lift and manoeuvre someone to avoid putting your back out and then being no good to anyone for weeks.

✔ **Have a flu jab every winter.** Even if your own ongoing health issues don't warrant this type of protection, because you care for someone you're eligible for the vaccination at your local GP surgery.

✔ **Don't neglect your own medical condition.** Have the relevant check-ups and blood tests when requested, see your dentist and optician for regular reviews and, if you're on any, make sure you keep taking the tablets.

If you don't like to 'bother' the doctor, a number of self-assessment tools are available on the NHS website (`www.nhs.uk/Tools/Pages/Wellbeing-self-assessment.aspx`) that allow you to give yourself a check-up. They're obviously not a substitute for seeing a clinical professional, but they act as a useful guide to whether you're as okay as you think you are or actually need to see a doctor. Be honest in your responses!

Remaining sane

Having a healthy body is worth little if your brain is all over the place. Being in the grip of depression or stressed out of your wits has a profound effect on your ability to care for someone else. Being a carer can take a mental as well as physical toll, so you need to take care of the precious organ inside your skull. You need it to stay sharp in order to do your job well. Again, staying fit, sleeping properly, eating well and not overdoing cigarettes or alcohol help you remain mentally robust. But being able to talk about issues and difficulties also helps prevent molehills developing into unconquerable mountains.

Many people see counselling as either hippy-dippy nonsense or reserved for those who've had a nervous breakdown. Neither of these stereotypes is true. First, talking therapies aren't nonsense; they can really help. Talking to trained professionals is better than chatting to family and friends, because they're both impartial and can offer guidance on dealing with unhelpful thought patterns. Second, psychotherapy and counselling aren't simply useful when you hit rock bottom; they can prevent you from getting that low in the first place. Talking to a therapist can help you get to know yourself better, identify your weak spots and pinpoint ways of thinking and behaving that can cause you trouble (and probably always have). By all means talk to your friends and family to help de-stress, but also seriously consider seeking out a professional therapist to help keep your mind healthy and your sanity intact. Your GP can recommend therapists and counsellors, some of whom may be funded by the NHS.

If you really can't stomach the idea of a face-to-face meeting with a therapist but would still like to stay in good mental health, consider reading a book on the subject. If you're not much of a reader, several excellent websites provide interactive tools for beating stress, anxiety and depression. I recommend Moodjuice (`www.moodjuice.scot.nhs.uk`) and MoodGYM (`https://moodgym.anu.edu.au/welcome`) to my patients.

Taking care of your spiritual health

Although the number of people attending a place of worship is apparently dwindling (only 6 per cent of the UK population do so, according to the 2011 census), surveys invariably show that far more people say they believe in God (34 per cent, according to a YouGov poll in the same year). If you're in either of those groups, or drift into them as life becomes a struggle (no atheists are present on the battlefield, they say), make sure you find a way to maintain your spiritual health too. Research findings presented by psychologist Roxanne Gervais in 2014 demonstrated that 'religiosity seemed to assist individuals in gaining better well-being and using more appropriate coping mechanisms'.

If you normally go to a church, mosque or temple, do your best to maintain that attendance. Also consider going on a religious or spiritual retreat to regain your equanimity or mental strength. If you can't leave the person with dementia for long enough to get to your place of worship, make every effort to stay in touch with other people who share your faith so that they can support you.

Approaching charities and support groups

A growing number of (mostly charitable) organisations help carers either directly by addressing their own needs or indirectly by looking after the person with dementia to give the carers a break. Some of these organisations are specifically related to dementia and others apply to all carers, whether they're looking after adults with dementia, children with disabilities or simply elderly relatives.

Dementia support

Organisations all over the UK offer support for people with dementia and their carers. Some are specific to a local area while others are centrally co-ordinated national organisations offering local provision.

An Internet search can give you an idea of what's around the corner, and the following list describes nationally run organisations that, even if they can't help you directly, can point you and the person you're caring for in the right direction:

✔ **Alzheimer's Society:** Based in England, Wales and Northern Ireland, it works to improve the quality of life of anyone affected by any of the main types of dementia. It provides more than 2,000 local services to support people with dementia and their carers, including memory cafes, group outings, specific carer support, and face-to-face, online and telephone sources of information on all aspects of dementia. Check out its website at www.alzheimers.org.uk or use the telephone helpline on 0300 222 1122.

✔ **Alzheimer's Scotland:** The Scottish-based cousin of the Alzheimer's Society, it provides similar support and information to that offered south of the border. Go to www.alzscot.org or use its free 24-hour helpline on 0808 808 3000.

✔ **Dementia UK:** This is another national charity aiming to improve the lives of all those with dementia, including their carers. It provides a great community service via its admiral nurses, specially trained mental health nurses with an interest in dementia. According to the Dementia UK website, admiral nurses

- Focus on the needs of the carer, including providing psychological support to help family carers understand and deal with their feelings.

- Help families better understand dementia and use a range of interventions that help people live well with the condition and develop skills to improve communication and maintain relationships.

- Are an invaluable source of contact and support for families at particular points of difficulty in the dementia journey, including diagnosis, when the condition advances and when tough decisions need to be made, such as moving a loved one into residential care.

- Provide advice on referrals to other appropriate services, and liaise with other healthcare professionals on behalf of the family.

Contact Dementia UK via its website (www.dementiauk.org) or direct helpline (0845 257 9406).

General support for carers

As well as specific support for those looking after people with dementia, generic support is also available for carers in general. You may be able to find local groups, but if not, the following are nationally run and open to all:

✔ **Carers Direct:** Although this NHS service doesn't offer emotional support for carers, it can direct you to the people in your area who do. It can also provide advice on pretty much everything you need to know as a carer, which may be stress-busting in itself.

According to the Carers Direct website, it offers information dealing with personal support needs and the needs of the person you're looking after, benefits, direct payments, individual budgets, and time off from, maintaining, leaving or going back to work or education. It also explains how to complain if anything goes wrong with the services you use, and can put you in touch with your local authority or NHS services.

Check out www.nhs.uk/carersdirect or use its free helpline on 0300 123 1053.

✔ **Carers UK:** This organisation is directly involved in supporting the estimated 6.5 million people in the UK who are unpaid volunteer carers. And this number is estimated to be rising by around 6,000 people every day.

Carers UK is the only national charity specifically dedicated to the needs of carers. According to its website, it

- Provides expert telephone advice, information and support on all aspects of the role of a carer, from claiming benefits and sorting out respite to accessing psychological emotional help

- Connects carers with each other locally and helps individual carers to join up with others through local support groups

- Is truly UK-wide, offering services in England, Wales, Scotland and Northern Ireland

Go to www.carersuk.org or use the telephone helpline on 0808 808 7777.

Asking for help from friends and family

Although for most people the traditional family model in which members live around the corner from each other is sadly a thing of the past, some extended families do still live in the same community. If that's the case for you, not only is accessing emotional support from siblings, cousins, aunts and uncles and even parents much easier, but so too is sharing the physical burden of caring.

Try to set up a rota of family members or close friends who can either pop in to visit the person with dementia every now and again or commit to caring for her on a particular day of the week. Not only does doing so give you a break – you can then get on with other things (or, better still, put your feet up) – but it also offers more stimulation for the person being cared for, because she gets a chance to interact with a wider circle of people instead of being stuck with the same old faces day in, day out.

Taking Time Out

When you work in a paid job, be it nine to five, shift work or some other arrangement, you expect to have breaks and holidays. Without them, both you and your bosses are well aware that your efficiency and productivity will suffer.

I always know when a holiday is overdue, because I become more easily stressed and irritated by small things and am perpetually tired. After some time off, I invariably return refreshed, invigorated and ready for whatever my patients and the NHS bosses throw at me.

Being a carer may be an unpaid job, but the stresses and pressures it presents are no less exhausting than those experienced by people in a paid occupation – if anything, they're worse. You thus need to ensure that you take some time out, and doing so is doubly important if you're still working as well as acting as a carer.

Acknowledging the importance of 'me time'

Making time for yourself each day is neither wrong nor inherently selfish. It needn't involve a trip to the local spa for a sauna, massage, pedicure and glass of bubbly, but it does mean making time for a bath full of bubbles, a potter in the greenhouse, a dip into a favourite novel, a wrestle with a crossword or Sudoku puzzle, or simply a stroll around the block.

I live with three lively teenage sons and often feel that the only time I get to myself is in the bathroom. And even then, and despite having another bathroom to choose from, I'm invariably interrupted by a call from outside to get a move on because someone else wants to get in. To make more time for myself, I now go for a run or a bike ride. I pop on my headphones, put my iPod on shuffle and spend a happy hour clearing my head before returning to the fray.

Spend your 'me time' doing something you enjoy – and make sure you do it every day.

Making time for tea

Interpret 'tea' as you will: the drink or the afternoon meal, alone or with friends. But whatever that word suggests to you, you need to make time for it.

We all know that when we're busy looking after someone else, our own basic needs can fall by the wayside; we can easily get to the end of the day hungry and thirsty because we've had nothing to eat or drink. As a carer, you need to ensure that you're fed and watered in order to be any good to the person you're looking after. Having a cuppa both provides an opportunity for rehydration and acts as a trigger to sit down for five minutes and take a breather. Making a cup of tea is also a task you can share with the person with dementia.

Going out for tea with friends is an even better way of getting some respite, whether you go alone or take the person with dementia with you. On your own with friends, it's a chance to get troubles off your chest or to have a laugh and forget about everything; together, it's a source of stimulation and different company.

Meeting friends

Friends can be your greatest source of moral and physical support, so staying in touch with them is very important. Unfortunately, if you're caring for someone 24 hours a day, cutting friends out of your life is all too easily done.

I have a patient in her 50s who still lives at home, because she looks after her dad who has vascular dementia. She does everything for him, from cooking meals to rinsing soiled underpants, and her life is tough. When she tries to go out he becomes upset and tearful and she responds by staying at home as he wants her to, becoming ever more isolated in the process.

Recently, however, an old school friend has begun popping around to see her every Tuesday evening for a couple of hours. Her dad's happy because she's at home, and she's happy because she gets a chance to share a couple of glasses of wine, reminisce about the old days, have a laugh and a cry and get things off her chest. That one evening a week has made a huge difference to her life.

Enjoying a hobby

As many different types of hobby exist as there are carers (well, almost), so finding something to tickle your fancy shouldn't be too difficult. Consider knitting, bowls, bird watching, cake baking, bridge or poker nights, tennis, swimming, dog walking – the list goes on.

You can take up a solitary hobby that allows you to simply enjoy time on your own, or you can engage in group hobbies that also provide an opportunity to meet new people and make friends. Choosing a hobby that you have to sign up to and pay for is even better, because you then feel duty-bound to attend. In effect, you're forced to take a break and have the psychological permission you need to leave your caring duties for a short while to go out and have fun.

Alongside the general benefits accruing from taking up a hobby and belonging to a group, a significant amount of research suggests that hobbies also increase a person's social capital. In simple terms, social capital refers to the collective and economic benefits that result when people co-operate in groups. Such groups can be closely interacting neighbours, members of clubs and societies, or people who belong to faith groups. Those with high social capital are demonstrably healthier, happier and less stressed.

So what have you got to lose? Whether you decide to take up a new hobby or re-engage in an old one, that activity can help keep you sane and fit enough to continue with your caring duties.

Getting away from it all

While short weekly breaks from the psychological and physical rigours of caring have obvious benefits, nothing quite beats downing tools for a week or two, packing a suitcase or backpack and getting away from it all. And whether that involves putting your feet up beside a pool in Spain, basking in the sun on a Greek island or donning your walking boots and exploring the South Downs in England doesn't matter; the prolonged period of time out is what's important.

Short breaks alone

Getting away on your own may well be a great way to recharge your batteries so that you can return to your caring role with more energy than you left it. You can choose from a whole range of short breaks in the UK and abroad, and some organisations actually provide breaks with carers in mind.

If you're a full-time carer for someone with dementia, you may be entitled to funding for a short break on your own. However, you may also have to organise the necessary interim care for the person you normally look after if family members can't step in. If you don't have the funds to secure the services of a privately recommended carer, the local council or various charities may help.

Respite care

To access local social services' help, you have to undergo a carer's assessment and the person you're looking after needs to have had a community care assessment (see Chapter 14). Both can be arranged through either your social worker if you have one, or through your local authority social services department if you don't. If you're stuck, your GP or specialist memory nurse can point you in the right direction.

Two types of respite care are available:

- **Residential or nursing care:** The person you're looking after enters a residential or nursing home for the duration of your holiday.

- **Day-sitting and night-sitting services:** Someone comes into your home during the day to care for the person you look after and is replaced by a night-sitter to cover the rest of the 24-hour period. This option is more often used when carers are spending part of a day or a night away from home. While it can work for a short break, especially if the person is better off in her own home, this type of care may need to be augmented by regular visits from friends and other family members.

Holidays together

You can also consider going away with the person you're looking after. This can work well particularly in the early stages of dementia if the person isn't too disabled by her symptoms. You have to do a lot of planning, however, to anticipate difficulties and find a way around them (borrowing a commode from the Red Cross, for example) to ensure the holiday is as relaxing and stress-free as possible. You don't want to spend the time desperate to get home for a rest.

Here are some tips from the Alzheimer's Society website (`www.alzheimers.org.uk`):

- Go on holiday with your extended family so that the caring tasks are shared among the group and you, as the main carer, still get some time out.

- Check out hotels in advance to ensure they're welcoming to someone with dementia, and warn them of the potential mishaps that could occur. Picking smaller hotels or B&Bs is a good idea, because fewer guests will be staying there and the building is less likely to have identical, and therefore confusing, corridors. Also check on disabled access and facilities, such as larger bathrooms and toilets, which make life easier too.

- Choose a holiday specifically designed for people with disabling conditions and their families. Vitalise (`www.vitalise.org.uk`) specialises in such breaks.

Sorting Out Your Own Finances

As a carer, particularly if you have lasting power of attorney, you're involved in making sure that your loved one's finances are in order. Making sure that you don't neglect your own finances is equally important, because you may still need to work, and you'll certainly have bills to pay.

With the possibility of your caring role expanding over time, you may well have to change your working pattern or even consider early retirement, and both situations have a potential knock-on effect on your income.

This section explores your options where your own employment is concerned, as well as looking at allowances you might be entitled to and whom to turn to for the best advice.

Changing to flexible working

You may need to alter your working arrangements if you're also acting as a carer for a person with dementia. 'Flexible working' is a legal term included in the Work and Families Act 2006. It covers alternative working patterns such as

- ✔ Flexi-time
- ✔ Staggered hours
- ✔ Compressed hours
- ✔ Working from home
- ✔ Job sharing

Under the terms of the act, those who care for other adults who are either spouses or close relatives can apply to alter their working hours. Employees can apply for flexible working if they've worked continuously for the same employer for the previous 26 weeks. Making a statutory application involves the following steps:

- ✔ The employee writes to the employer detailing her reasons for applying for flexible working arrangements; alternatively, she can download a form from www.gov.uk/flexible-working/overview, fill it in and present that to her employer.

- ✔ The employer considers the request and has to make a decision within three months, unless a longer period of consideration is agreed with the employee.

- ✔ If the employer agrees to the request, it must change the terms and conditions in the employee's contract, and the process is complete.

- ✔ If the employer disagrees, it must write to the employee citing the business reasons for the refusal. The employee may be able to present her case to an employment tribunal to try to reverse that decision.

You can make one application for flexible working per year.

Understanding retirement and pensions

When you reach retirement age, you're eligible for your state pension plus income from any private or business pensions you may have, such as those provided by the NHS, armed forces and civil service. Retirement age is currently 65 for men and 60 for women; however, these are set to rise to 65 for women by November 2018, and 66 for both men and women by November 2020. As a carer, you will be able to collect your spouse's pension if you have lasting power of attorney.

If you're still working but have to cut your hours in order to take on a caring role for more than 20 hours per week then the government will top up your National Insurance contributions via what's called carer's credit, to ensure you still receive your full pension entitlement when you reach retirement age. For more information see www.gov.uk/carers-credit.

Applying for carer's allowance

In addition to any earnings or income from pensions, you may be able to apply for a carer's allowance. To be eligible, you must meet these criteria:

✔ You must be 16 years old or over.

✔ You must look after someone for at least 35 hours a week.

✔ The person you look after must receive a qualifying disability benefit.

✔ If you work, you must not have net earnings above £100 a week.

✔ You must be living in the UK when you claim carer's allowance, and satisfy certain residence and immigration rules.

✔ You must not be a full-time student.

Your eligibility won't be affected by any savings you've accumulated. Visit www.gov.uk for more details.

Taking financial advice

Whenever your life circumstances change – for example, when you get a job, get married or become a carer – asking an independent financial adviser to review your finances is a good idea. Not only can a financial adviser make sure that your savings and insurance policies are in order, but she can also identify whether you're receiving all that you're entitled to. Use the advice offered to make sure that you can cope financially in your new circumstances.

Go to www.unbiased.co.uk to find an independent financial advisor – the name says it all!

Being a 'good enough' carer

No one's super-human; we can only ever do our best. Although this revelation shouldn't be seen as an excuse to drop your standards, it's none-theless reassuring to know that being 'good enough' still means you're doing a good job.

British paediatrician and psychoanalyst Donald Winnicott (1896–1971) developed the concept of 'good enough' during his work with mothers and their babies in the 1950s. He wanted to reassure these women that failing sometimes is fine and striving for perfection is merely frustrating. For Winnicott, a 'good enough' mother does her best to give her baby appropriate attention, physical care and emotional support, and cre-ates a safe environment in which her child can develop independence. She's not a quitter, and when she fails at something, which she inevita-bly does, she gets right back in the saddle and gives it another go. In short, she demonstrates a sacrificial love that makes allowances for get-ting things wrong. This concept allows mums to acknowledge feeling resentful about the stress of their role and having to put their own needs to one side in order to look after their baby, all for very little thanks. It also allows them to be annoyed with their baby at times without subse-quently feeling that they're bad mothers.

This concept can clearly be applied to every-one who has a hands-on role as a carer. Carers can never perform the role perfectly, and at times they'll feel angry, frustrated and resentful. They'll do some things badly and forget to do others. But most of the time, their desire to do their best means that things will be fine and the person they're looking after will be safe and well cared for and know that she's loved.

If you're a carer for someone with dementia, take Dr Winnicott's wisdom on board and rec-ognise that being a 'good enough' carer is good enough.

Chapter 13

Sourcing Help: Working Your Way Around the System

In This Chapter

▶ Identifying who's who in the NHS and where to find them

▶ Recognising what social services departments have to offer

▶ Getting help from dementia charities and voluntary organisations

*B*eing passed from pillar to post and from department to department is the last thing you need when you're in a difficult situation and seeking help. It's intensely frustrating and also increases your feeling of helplessness. When you're knee-deep in the many physical, social and psychological difficulties that dementia involves, you need to feel supported and that you have somewhere to turn for help.

Fortunately, a whole host of professionals working in the NHS, social services and the voluntary sector will be only too pleased to step in and give you the support you need, from first diagnosis to the final stages of the disease. In this chapter I take a look at who these people are, where you can find them, and what sort of services they can offer both you and the person you're caring for.

Starting at the Doctor's Surgery

Your local doctor's surgery or health centre is likely to be your first port of call when seeking help. Here's a guide to the different professionals based there and their roles.

General practitioners

General practitioners (GPs) are the gateway to most of the treatments and services that are available on the NHS. As part of an integrated primary healthcare team, a GP has a finger in many pies and can signpost you to services run by other bodies such as local-authority social-care departments and charitable and voluntary organisations. Not only is a GP your first port of call when you're worried about a diagnosis, but he'll also be able to adapt his approach as things progress, and can put you in touch with the most relevant people to help at each stage.

Some practices have a GP with a special interest in dementia. This fact is probably advertised in the practice leaflet or on its website. If not, ask the receptionist whether the practice has such a GP.

In many ways, though, continuity of care with the GP who knows the dementia patient best may be ideal. The usual GP knows the patient's background and is therefore better placed to observe any changes than is a GP who has just become involved. The existing GP can also continue to monitor other, more longstanding conditions the patient may have.

To ensure you get the most from the initial appointment with the GP:

- ✔ Try to see the person's usual GP and ask for a double appointment. Most appointments are only around 12 minutes long, which won't be enough.
- ✔ Think about what you want to get from the appointment before you go.
- ✔ Write down a list of questions so that you don't forget anything.
- ✔ List any symptoms that are causing concern, so that they can be addressed.
- ✔ If tests are suggested, ask what they involve, how long they'll take and how soon the results will be available.
- ✔ Ask whether referral to a specialist memory clinic is available or appropriate.
- ✔ See what local services are available, such as clubs and support for carers.
- ✔ Discuss what you can do to keep yourself healthy.
- ✔ Find out about how to get in touch with social services and what they can provide in terms of support and home adaptations.

If, for whatever reason, you don't get on with your GP, you can either change to another GP within the practice or change surgeries altogether. You can simply turn up at a different practice armed with your NHS medical card and fill in a registration form. Your medical notes will then be transferred to the new GP – no questions asked.

While your GP may be aware that you or someone you love has dementia, he's not psychic and doesn't automatically know when things aren't going well or new symptoms have developed. Keep in touch with him so that he can offer help as soon as it's needed.

Practice nurses

Most GP practices in the UK have at least one practice nurse, who offers a variety of services. Practice nurses tend to offer longer appointments than GPs do, so they can often cover things in more detail. You can book an appointment with the practice nurse directly at your surgery's reception, or you may be referred by your GP. The practice nurse's role includes

- ✔ Carrying out general health checks, monitoring things like blood pressure and weight, and taking routine blood tests
- ✔ Giving general health and lifestyle advice, particularly in relation to diet and exercise
- ✔ Reviewing long-term medication; specifically, checking for side effects and that pills are still doing their job

Some nurses are able to prescribe medication and may run minor illness clinics for treating simple chest or urinary-tract infections. The practice receptionist can direct you to the most appropriate nurse.

Checking Out Community-Based Services

These services aren't attached to a particular GP surgery, but their staff cover a number of practices in a local area so that their skills and expertise can be shared. Community-based services see people in their own homes and are usually accessed via the GP.

Community matrons

Community matrons are highly skilled and experienced senior nurses who work as case managers. They're generally responsible for around 50 patients with complex medical needs. Community matrons are able to do the following:

- ✔ Carry out physical examinations.
- ✔ Decide on treatment, and issue prescriptions.

✔ Arrange for tests such as urine and blood tests.

✔ Refer patients to hospital clinics, specialists or other professionals such as physiotherapists and occupational therapists.

✔ Carry out follow-ups to ensure continuity of care.

✔ Visit their patients when they're in hospital to help work out safe and effective discharge plans.

Community matrons are a wonderful addition to the primary healthcare team and play a vital role in enabling vulnerable people to remain in their own homes, when it's safe to do so. They work closely with GPs in order to facilitate this arrangement.

Community nurses for older people

Like matrons, this group of nurses works out and about in the community, visiting people in their own homes. They work closely with GPs and community matrons. The community nurse's role includes

✔ Providing health education

✔ Monitoring patients with long-term conditions to check for deterioration

✔ Assessing evolving health needs

✔ Signposting patients to other services

✔ Providing advice on long-term care options such as residential homes, warden-controlled flats and nursing-home placements

You can access community nurses for older people via a GP, but they also accept direct referrals from friends, family members and carers.

District nurses

Although, sadly, district nurses no longer peddle around on bicycles administering to the sick and wounded, their skills are just as evident in the 21st century. Maybe they're in even better shape now that being saddle sore isn't an issue!

District nurses are part of the primary-care team and usually cover a number of different GP practices from a central base. A district nurse can often be contacted directly or by referral from your GP, and can help with the following care needs:

✔ Changing dressings

✔ Treating wounds and bed sores

✔ Monitoring progress at home after hospital discharge

✔ Giving injections

✔ Offering general healthcare advice

✔ Providing end-of-life care

Homing in on Hospital-Based Services

Your GP can refer people to a number of specialist healthcare professionals based in hospital clinics. In the following sections I describe the hospital-based healthcare professionals that you're most likely to come across.

Specialist dementia or memory nurses

These nurses, as their name suggests, are trained specifically to help with the care needs of people with dementia. They may work in secondary-care hospital clinics, in primary care in the community or in a mixture of both settings. In some areas of the country they are called admiral nurses, and sadly in some areas these nurses do not yet exist.

Specialist dementia nurses carry out detailed tests to diagnose whether a person has dementia and to differentiate between the types of dementia (see Chapter 3 for more on this). These nurses also help families to understand the condition better, and provide information on sources of help.

Dementia nurses work closely with specialist doctors and can arrange for people whose symptoms are deteriorating to be reviewed. They can also advise GPs on changes in medication. Dementia nurses often work closely with GP surgeries and become involved in a person's care via a GP referral.

Hospital consultants

Hospital consultants are doctors with extensive training in a specific area. Depending on where you live and the age of the person with dementia, you may deal with one or all of the following specialists:

✔ **Psychiatrists:** These doctors work with people with a variety of mental health problems.

✔ **Old-age psychiatrists:** These psychiatrists deal with the particular mental health issues experienced by people over the age of 65.

✔ **Neurologists:** These specialists treat conditions of the brain and nervous system, and may often be needed to help diagnose dementia in a younger person when the symptoms are not clear cut.

✔ **Geriatricians (or care-of-the-elderly physicians):** Geriatricians are doctors with expertise in treating physical diseases that occur particularly in old age.

Consultants can't be accessed directly, but GPs can refer patients for appointments. Because consultants work in teams with more junior doctors and specialist nurses, your appointment may be with any of these professionals.

Considering Other Health Professionals

Focusing on a chronic condition like dementia that affects a person in so many ways can mean a carer forgets to also consider that person's general health. People with dementia may have arthritis, cataracts and poor hearing, just like everyone else, and leaving these problems untreated can dramatically add to their disability.

Mobility specialists

Mobility is often an issue for elderly people, whether or not they have dementia. Maintaining muscle strength and flexibility is vital for this, and taking care of your feet can make a big difference to your quality of life if you have dementia. The two specialists you're likely to encounter are

✔ **Physiotherapists:** Physiotherapists work both for the NHS and in private practice. They can treat pain and immobility resulting from arthritis, help mobilise someone after a fracture or joint surgery, and provide exercises to help improve stability and prevent falls. While they generally work in hospital departments, many physiotherapists also treat people at home.

✔ **Podiatrists:** These foot specialists, also known as chiropodists, play a vital role in keeping feet healthy and pain free. They can treat a wide variety of problems from simple corns and ingrowing toenails to bunions. Like physiotherapists, they're available with a GP referral on the NHS but may also work in private practice.

Ear, teeth and eye specialists

Again, just like everyone else, people with dementia may experience problems with their hearing, teeth and eyesight. And with dementia in particular, it's important that people can make full use of their senses. It's easy to think someone is not remembering when he simply didn't hear what was said. Dealing with these issues will improve someone's general wellbeing.

These are some of the specialists who can help:

✔ **Audiologists:** Poor hearing is disabling enough on its own, but when combined with the symptoms of dementia it can lead to increasing confusion and isolation. Hearing checks are vital, but may well need to be preceded by a trip to the practice nurse at the GP surgery to ensure that a build-up of wax isn't the simple culprit.

✔ **Dentists:** These professionals aren't everyone's favourite, and a visit to the dentist can become increasingly difficult as dementia and its associated confusion progresses. It's a good idea for people with dementia to have regular dental checks with a dentist they already know to ensure they have healthy teeth and gums. Some dentists can also arrange home visits.

✔ **Opticians/optometrists:** As people get older, a multitude of eye conditions, from cataracts to macular degeneration, can gang up and affect the eyesight. As with hearing difficulties, the sensory deprivation resulting from poor eyesight worsens symptoms of confusion, so regular eye tests are vital.

Seeking Help from Social Services

Good social care and support is as vital in dementia as any of the services the NHS can provide. A person with dementia may not become unwell, and may remain as fit as a fiddle physically, never needing to darken the doctor's door. But it's rare that someone with dementia won't eventually have difficulties with what the professionals call activities of daily living, such as

✔ Cooking

✔ Cleaning

✔ Shopping

✔ Washing

✔ Dressing

✔ Dealing with money

Social services can come in very handy here.

Who's who?

You might need to be in touch with two types of social service professional to organise a care plan and to sort out adaptations to make life easier for the person with dementia:

- ✔ **Social workers:** Are qualified to assess your care needs and plan services for you. They help to arrange home care needs, respite and moves into residential care. They also provide advice on other community services.

- ✔ **Occupational therapists:** Carry out home assessments to advise on adaptations that can help you to maintain independence. They'll sort out hand rails and walk-in showers, for example.

How do you get hold of them?

Every local authority has a social care department that takes referrals directly from relatives and carers as well as from GPs and nurses. You can find details on the local authority's website or in the *Yellow Pages*.

Is Anybody Else Out There?

Services exist to help with pretty much all the difficulties that people with dementia and their carers may experience:

- ✔ **Day centres:** These centres provide help and support, involve people in physically and mentally stimulating activities such as games and crafts, and provide opportunities to meet other people.

- ✔ **Home adaptations:** Social services can help make people's homes safer for them to live in by providing hand rails, walk-in showers, raised toilet seats and outside access ramps.

- ✔ **Home help:** A home help can provide assistance with getting in and out of bed, dressing, cooking, cleaning, shopping and bathing.

- ✔ **Meals on wheels:** This service, run by volunteers, delivers hot, nutritious meals every day, seven days a week if needed.

- ✔ **Personal alarms:** Worn on the wrist or around the neck, these alarms connect to a control centre. If someone falls, for example, the control centre can contact a relative or call an ambulance.

My sister is a district nurse and has encountered people with dementia who live in a house with an alarm. If the person opens the front door in the night, for example, the alarm alerts a relative or control centre. Alarms can also detect that the cooker has been left on.

✔ **Respite care:** A short period in a care home can give older people living on their own a break, and can also give carers time to recharge their batteries.

Checking Out Charities and the Voluntary Sector

People in the UK are very fortunate to have a variety of charities that support not only people with dementia but, just as importantly, their carers too. These charities provide a wide range of services, such as

✔ Advocacy services

✔ Befriending schemes

✔ Day centres

✔ Dementia advisors and support workers

✔ Memory cafes

✔ Specialist nurses

✔ Support groups for people with dementia and their carers

You can find out more from the organisations themselves, details of which are listed in Appendix A. But to give you a flavour of what's on offer, I give a few examples of the services mentioned.

Befriending schemes

Befrienders are volunteers who regularly visit people with dementia to help encourage social contact by chatting, playing games, listening to music together, or getting out and about for short trips for afternoon tea or simply to get a breath of fresh air.

Befrienders also, of course, take the strain off carers for a while so they can get on with things they wouldn't otherwise be able to do around the house or, even better, just chill out and grab a moment or two for themselves.

Memory cafes

Memory cafes have sprung up all over the UK as places where people with any memory-related problems, but particularly dementia, can enjoy a break from their normal routine by meeting other people and having a piece of cake and a good old-fashioned cup of tea in a relaxing, supportive environment. Carers, too, can hang out with other carers and share stories, hints and tips, and generally support one another.

Cafes are staffed by volunteers whose aim is to provide companionship and reminiscence therapy and encourage people to join in with communal games. They're also available to give advice and support to carers.

Support groups

Carers of people with dementia invariably carry a heavy burden, which is often made even harder by a sense of guilt. Although it's rarely justified, guilt does seem to come with the territory, either because carers think they should be capable of more or because they regret moments of anger and irritability. They also have little time for themselves, to look after their own health, see friends, indulge in hobbies or simply get some well-earned rest.

Support groups for carers offer advice, provide signposts to other services and offer a listening ear when it all gets a bit much. They're available around the UK and can often be contacted by phone or email.

Nothing's wrong with asking for help. Most carers are unpaid family members and not trained professionals. They're not supposed to know everything or to cope alone with what can be very difficult circumstances. If you're in that position, bear in mind that if you become ill yourself because you don't get the help you need, your loved one may then have no one to care for him.

Chapter 14

Sorting Out Benefits

· ·

In This Chapter

▶ Considering welfare benefits that can help people with dementia

▶ Working through the application process

▶ Understanding how to appeal if your application is turned down

· ·

*H*aving the right level of care when you have dementia doesn't come cheaply. And the amount of work family members put in as non-professional carers is not without its costs either, no matter how much it's motivated by love.

Fortunately, to help with the cost of care, some government benefits are available for both dementia sufferers and their carers. Many of the benefits are financially means tested.

In this chapter I look at the benefits available, how to access them and who can assist you in making sure you're not missing out on any much-needed help that you're entitled to. I start with a rundown of which benefits you can apply for.

Knowing Which Benefits Are Available

Read the headlines in some of the UK's national tabloid newspapers and you'll think that the benefits system is just a way for scroungers and idlers to earn an easy buck from the comfort of their brand new, reclining sofas without having to lift a finger. Most recipients are either undeserving layabouts or immigrants who've exploited loopholes in the system to get their hands on honest taxpayers' money. But this simply isn't true.

We should be proud of the welfare state, of which benefits are a part. The system ensures that the most vulnerable people in our society can receive decent care and provision. Unfortunately, the stigma that the braying headlines generates puts many people off applying for benefits to which they're entitled, because they fear they'll be labelled as scroungers themselves.

Applying for benefits is nothing to be ashamed of: they're there to help when you find yourself or a loved one in need, and they're financed by the taxes you and your family have already paid while able to work. Don't struggle unnecessarily.

The founding father of the modern welfare state was economist Sir William Beveridge, whose report for the coalition government of 1942 identified 'five giant evils' of society: want, squalor, idleness, ignorance and disease. The report recommended a flat-rate insurance scheme that would cover ill-health, unemployment and retirement.

When the Labour Party won the general election in 1945, it began to put Beveridge's recommendation into practice with the intention of providing for the nation's sick and vulnerable 'from the cradle to the grave'. And although some subsequent governments have squeezed how much of the national purse is spent on providing for these members of society, a fairly extensive system of welfare benefits is still available to those deemed to qualify for support.

Currently, three main types of benefits are directly related to disability. They aim to

✔ Cover the extra cost of meeting care and mobility needs.

✔ Replace lost earnings.

✔ Top up earnings if someone is on a low income.

I cover specific benefits in the following sections.

Care and mobility benefits

Different benefits are available for people in different age categories; the benefits vary depending on whether the person with dementia is aged 16 to 64 or 65 and over. The benefits are also different depending on where in the UK someone lives.

Personal Independence Payment and Disability Living Allowance

The Personal Independence Payment (PIP) is gradually replacing the Disability Living Allowance (DLA). (In Northern Ireland, the benefit is still called Disability Living Allowance.) PIP is a tax-free benefit payable every four weeks to people aged 16 to 64, whether they're still in work or not. It doesn't depend on levels of savings or whether people have ever paid National Insurance contributions.

PIP has two components, and a person's entitlement to one or both depends on her illness and the results of an initial assessment of her needs. The two components are awarded at standard and enhanced rates and, according to the government's website (www.gov.uk), cover the following:

- ✔ **Daily living component:** This benefit is for people who need help with preparing or eating food, washing, bathing and using the toilet, dressing and undressing, reading and communicating, managing medication or treatments, making decisions about money and engaging with other people.

- ✔ **Mobility component:** As its name suggests, this benefit is for those who have trouble getting out and about and moving around, and for people who necessitate supervision from at least one other.

To qualify for either component of the PIP, a person must have experienced the difficulties for at least three months and expect them to last for at least nine months. These needs will be reassessed regularly.

Attendance Allowance

This benefit is available for people over the age of 65. It's a payment to help with care needs and, like PIP, is divided into two rates – lower and higher – depending on the level of care needed:

- ✔ **Lower rate:** This rate is awarded to people who need significant or constant supervision during *either* the day or the night.

- ✔ **Higher rate:** People who qualify for this rate need care *throughout* the day and night, or are terminally ill.

Unlike the PIP, Attendance Allowance doesn't include a mobility component.

Benefits for carers

A Carer's Allowance is paid to people who provide regular and substantial care to people in their homes. Carers don't have to be family members but must fit the following stringent criteria:

- ✔ Be over age 16 and not in full-time education.

- ✔ Spend at least 35 hours per week caring for someone who's in receipt of Attendance Allowance, the daily living component of the PIP or the personal care rate of the DLA.

- ✔ Not have a net income of more than £100 per week.

- ✔ Have been resident in the UK for two out of the previous three years.

Work and retirement benefits

Benefits are available to provide financial assistance to people who are under retirement age and not fit to work *or* who've reached retirement age but haven't been able to work for long enough to secure a full state pension.

Employment and Support Allowance

Employment and Support Allowance (ESA) is for people under retirement age who've been forced to stop work as a result of ill health or disability or who don't qualify for statutory sick pay. ESA has two categories: one for those who've paid sufficient National Insurance contributions during their working lives (contributory ESA), and one for those whose incomes and earnings are low (income-related ESA).

Some people qualify for both ESA categories but, like for all benefits, have to undergo official checks to confirm genuine eligibility.

State pension and pension credit

In response to an ageing population, the government has raised the age at which you're entitled to receive a state pension. Currently, the retirement age is 65 for men and 60 for women born before 4 May 1950. By 2020 it will be 66 for both men and women, and after that it will rise to 68.

In order to qualify for a full state pension you need to have paid 30 years' worth of National Insurance contributions. If you're entitled to a state pension, the Pension Service will contact you directly four months before you can start claiming it.

If you're not entitled to a full state pension, you may be able to claim Pension Credit, which tops up your weekly income. Surprise surprise, this benefit involves two elements: guarantee credit and savings credit. *Guarantee credit* tops up the pension to a guaranteed level; *savings credit* is calculated on the basis of someone's additional income from any savings. You may be entitled to claim for both.

Understanding How to Claim

Despite offering this extensive set of benefits, governments of all political persuasions are notoriously keen to hold on to as much of the allotted cash as possible. Obviously, this is the case because the government wants to ensure that recipients are truly deserving and that enough is in the collective pot to provide for everyone who qualifies.

As a result of this caution, people have to jump through a number of hoops in order to claim any of the benefits described in the preceding section. Some of these hoops involve filling in paper or online forms; others take the form of a face-to-face, independent medical assessment.

Knowing whom to contact

If you're technologically savvy and have access to the Internet, a good place to start is the government's benefits website at www.gov.uk. Here you can find details of all available benefits, the full application criteria, a description of the assessment process and forms to download. The website also gives a number to call to discuss any queries further or to use to make applications directly over the phone.

If you're not computer literate and prefer your communication via the postal service, I provide a list of contact addresses in Appendix A at the end of this book. Other sources of information include your local Citizens Advice branch and charities such as the Alzheimer's Society and Age UK.

Accessing the right forms

For all the benefits described in this chapter, you'll encounter forms to complete. They can often be quite lengthy documents asking in-depth questions about all the ways in which your dementia affects you.

After you've submitted your form, the Department for Work and Pensions (DWP) may send another set of paperwork to your GP, asking more detailed questions about health, the treatment received and the way in which your doctor feels the symptoms of dementia are affecting you. You don't have to see your GP in relation to this form; she'll simply fill it in based on what's recorded in your medical notes and from her knowledge of you.

You can apply for some benefits over the phone, avoiding writer's cramp altogether. Check www.gov.uk for details.

Getting help with your application

If you have to fill out a form to apply for your particular benefit, do seek help. Too many people are put off by the complicated appearance of these documents and thus don't bother to apply; as a result, they miss out on financial help that they're not only entitled to but could also really do with.

Cynics say that the DWP makes these forms as complicated as possible because it wants to keep hold of its money. To compound the problem, we Brits tend to adopt a stiff-upper-lip approach to answering the questions on the forms, often playing down the severity of our symptoms so as not to look like we're making a fuss. To ensure the best chance of success with your application, therefore, get some help from someone who can not only make sense of what's being asked but also make sure you give honest answers.

Family members may well be a good initial source of help, or you may have a friend or neighbour who's skilled in administrative matters and whom you don't mind knowing about your business. If you want impartial, independent help with deciphering what information the application forms are after and filling them in in a way that gives you the best chance of success, however, a number of organisations are available to help.

Citizens Advice

Citizens Advice is a national organisation with offices all over the UK. It offers free, impartial, independent and confidential advice on all aspects of people's rights and responsibilities. This advice is available online via the websites of individual Citizens Advice offices, over the phone or face to face from advisers. Some Citizens Advice offices even provide home visits and advice by email.

Volunteers who are well versed in the ins and outs of the benefit system and the intricacies of filling out the application forms staff the Citizens Advice offices. When you book an appointment, an adviser will tell you what information the organisation needs to know in order to help with your claim. As a guide, the main Citizens Advice website (www.citizensadvice.org.uk) suggests that you bring the following documents and information:

- Birth certificate
- National Insurance number
- Any payslips or details of benefits you already receive
- Bank statements
- Details of savings
- Mortgage payments or tenancy agreement
- Council tax bill
- And, of course, the forms you'd like help completing

The adviser may also ask you to provide more information about your health. If you provide written consent, the Citizens Advice adviser can contact your GP directly.

Charities

A number of the UK charities specifically involved in the care of people with dementia, or elderly people in general, offer help with claiming benefits and filling in forms. If a charity isn't able to help you directly, it can direct you to organisations in your area that can help.

You can contact the following organisations:

- Age UK
- Alzheimer's Society
- Carers Trust
- Carers UK

Contact details for all these charities can be found in Appendix A.

To help in preparing your application, these charities will probably need you to supply the documents and information listed in the 'Citizens Advice' section.

Challenging a decision you're unhappy with

If you have a query about or disagree with a decision that's been made in relation to your benefit application, you can take a number of different steps. To stand even a reasonable chance of success, your appeal has to be made through the correct channels and in a clearly specified way.

All the benefits related to dementia are provided by the DWP. The following sections describe the appeal process for this government department. (Other departments have their own specific procedures to follow.)

Mandatory reconsideration

For all appeals, you must first ask the DWP to reconsider its decision. After you've received a letter informing you of the DWP's decision, you have one calendar month in which to ask for the decision to be reconsidered. You can do so by phone or letter – there's no form to fill in. Citizens Advice advises sending a letter and keeping a copy for your records. The DWP's initial letter will tell you where to send your request.

Obtaining help with end-of-life care

Special rules apply to end-of-life care that allow people to receive the maximum in benefits as soon as possible. You need to see your GP for help in completing the necessary paperwork: form DS1500.

Completion of this form allows rapid payment of PIP or Attendance Allowance to anyone who's suffering with a progressive disease and not expected to live beyond a further six months. The person herself can make the claim or, as more often happens in the case of dementia,

someone can claim on her behalf. Bear in mind that because the prognosis cannot be exact, the benefit doesn't cease being paid once six months has elapsed.

A GP, consultant or specialist nurse must confirm the terminal nature of the illness on the DS1500 form. When you send off the form, you need to apply for PIP or Attendance Allowance at the same time. Then, as soon as the DS1500 is accepted, the application process is accelerated and prompt payment assured.

A different decision maker at the DWP from the one who considered your application usually looks at your claim. If this person thinks your claim is unlikely to succeed without new supporting evidence, she'll phone you to discuss it or write if she's unable to get hold of you. You then have a further month in which to provide new or extra evidence.

Once the DWP has reconsidered its decision, you'll either receive backdated payment of the benefit if you're successful, or the original decision will be upheld. In the latter case, you then have the right to appeal.

Appeals process

Appeals are lodged with the HM Courts and Tribunal Service rather than with the DWP. You lodge an appeal by filling in form SSCS1. You'll receive this form in the post, together with an accompanying booklet about how to fill it in.

As with the initial application, you're more likely to be successful in your appeal if you have professional help in filling out the form. In technical parlance, this person is called your *representative*. Although she can be a friend or family member, she does need to be able to help in the following ways:

- ✔ Advise you on the evidence you need to prepare to help you with your case.
- ✔ Help you to get this evidence.
- ✔ Be prepared to talk to the DWP to see whether it can change the decision in your favour without going to a tribunal.
- ✔ Research the law.
- ✔ Prepare a written statement for the tribunal hearing.

✔ Advise you on other benefits or legal help you may be entitled to.

✔ Help you with anything you need to do after the tribunal hearing.

If no one you know can help in this process, approach Citizens Advice.

You have only one month in which to appeal, so don't drag your heels.

You'll be given a date for the appeal hearing, which you can attend yourself if you want to. You can also take witnesses if you think they'll help. The tribunal decides whether to uphold the DWP's decision or overturn it, depending on the evidence that you provide.

Chapter 15

Addressing Legal Issues

A diagnosis of dementia gives you and your family a chance to plan for the future. So while your head will still no doubt be in a complete spin just taking in the fact that you have dementia and what that may mean to you and your family medically and physically over the coming months and years, it's important also to make plans about the more practical side of your life to avoid any problems later with care or finances. Doing so as early as possible, while you're still able to make decisions for yourself, is an excellent idea.

Setting Up an Advance Directive (a Living Will)

An *advance directive*, the more technical term for what many of us call a living will, is a document that allows you to indicate the types of medical treatment you would refuse under certain circumstances in the future, if at the time you're no longer either to make this decision for yourself or to communicate it to others.

In legal parlance, an advance directive allows your wishes to be respected if at any time you 'lack capacity'. Decisions about capacity are based on the Mental Capacity Act 2005.

Understanding the Mental Capacity Act

This act aims to empower and protect all vulnerable people when they're no longer able to make important decisions for themselves. Its underlying principle, according to the UK's Ministry of Justice, is 'to ensure that those who lack capacity are empowered to make as many decisions for themselves as possible and that any decision made, or action taken, on their behalf is made in their best interests'.

In order to try to achieve this outcome for vulnerable people, the act has five key principles (sourced from www.justice.gov.uk):

- ✔ Every adult has the right to make his own decisions and must be assumed to have capacity to make them unless it's proved otherwise. Therefore the onus is on the assessor to prove the individual lacks capacity, not the individual to prove he has it.

- ✔ A person must be given all practicable help before anyone treats him as not being able to make his own decisions.

- ✔ Just because an individual makes what may be seen as an unwise decision, he should not be treated as lacking capacity to make that decision.

- ✔ Anything done or any decision made on behalf of a person who lacks capacity must be done in his best interests.

- ✔ Anything done for or on behalf of a person who lacks capacity should be the least restrictive of his basic rights and freedoms.

This law is obviously intended to protect people with a range of different underlying medical problems, such as brain tumours, strokes, severe depression, schizophrenia or learning disabilities. But it's also important for people with dementia.

Defining 'capacity'

The law deems that people who lack capacity cannot do any or all of the following:

- ✔ Understand information given to them.
- ✔ Must have an impairment.
- ✔ Retain information long enough to be able to make a decision.
- ✔ Weigh up the information available to make a decision.
- ✔ Communicate their decision.

Assessment of capacity is decision specific. In other words, no one can make a once-and-for-all decision that someone is now and will always be completely incapable of making decisions about things that affect him. An assessment has to be made on a case-by-case basis, looking at one particular issue at one specific time only. This situation exists because a person with dementia, for example, may not be capable of making decisions about managing his money, but may be able to very clearly state that he'd like his appendix removed when he's in severe pain as a result of appendicitis.

Assessing capacity

A person's doctor (GP or specialist) usually makes an assessment of capacity in consultation with the person's family and main carers. During the assessment, the doctor does his best to communicate the issues at stake to give the person the best chance of getting to grips with the situation and its ramifications. The doctor then tries to establish whether, on the balance of probabilities, the person lacks the ability to make the particular decision because he's unable to understand, retain and weigh up the information he's just been given and then effectively communicate it.

Defining 'best interests'

If a person is deemed to lack capacity, any decision or action taken on his behalf must be in his best interests. These decisions will be made by a *decision maker*, who's usually the person's main carer, doctor or social worker, and must conform to the following guidelines:

- ✔ The person who lacks capacity must be involved.
- ✔ The decision maker must be aware of the person's wishes and feelings.
- ✔ Consultation must occur with others who are involved in the care of the person.
- ✔ No assumptions should be made based solely on the person's age, appearance, condition or behaviour.
- ✔ Consideration must be given to whether the person is likely to regain capacity to make the decision in the future.

Recognising what an advance directive can cover

An advance directive helps you to be one step ahead of the game in relation to losing capacity, because it enables you to decide what will or will not be in your best interests if certain important decisions need to be made. These decisions will therefore be made *by* you and not *for* you.

Examples of such decisions include your wishes regarding life-saving treatment such as

- ✔ Cardiopulmonary resuscitation
- ✔ Intensive care treatment
- ✔ Blood transfusions
- ✔ Antibiotics and intravenous fluids

Your decisions expressed in an advance directive are legally binding, thus any doctors involved in your care have to uphold them.

An advance directive cannot, however, be used by you to

- ✔ Specify treatments that you *do* want.
- ✔ Refuse treatment of severe mental health conditions.
- ✔ Request illegal treatments such as assisted suicide.
- ✔ Refuse basic care and hygiene to keep you comfortable.
- ✔ Refuse food and drink.

While you still have capacity, your word overrides anything written in an advance directive.

Getting hold of the paperwork

Some organisations working with people with dementia, such as the Alzheimer's Society, or with terminal illnesses, for example Macmillan, provide downloadable example advance directive forms on their websites. But you don't need to complete an official document. If you're preparing an advance directive for yourself, you must include the following details:

- ✔ Your name, date of birth and address
- ✔ The name, address and phone number of your GP, and whether he has a copy of your advance directive document
- ✔ A statement making clear that this advance directive document should be used if you ever lack capacity to make decisions
- ✔ A statement regarding which treatment(s) you will refuse, and the circumstances in which your decision will apply
- ✔ The date you created your advance directive
- ✔ Your signature
- ✔ A dated signature of at least one witness

If you're writing an advance directive to refuse medical treatment that will keep you alive, it must also include the statement, 'I refuse this treatment even if my life is at risk as a result.'

Talking through possible scenarios with your GP as you draw up your document and before putting pen to paper and signing it is always best. Your doctor can help you understand what you may face in certain circumstances, and what refusal of treatment will mean in terms of the symptoms you may therefore suffer and the effect on your life expectancy.

Examples of statements covering scenarios you may want to include after this discussion are

- ✔ 'I refuse artificial feeding and rehydrating fluids, even if my life is at risk as a result, if I have terminal cancer and become unconscious and unable to eat or drink without assistance.'

- ✔ 'If I have a condition from which I'm expected to die in a matter of days or weeks, I only want treatment to help manage discomfort and distress and not to prolong my life, even if my life is at risk as a result.'

You should review your advance directive with family, carers and your doctor at regular intervals, because it can be rescinded or altered at any time in the light of changing circumstances.

Identifying which professionals to involve

You'll probably be pleased to learn that, unless you really want to, you don't have to involve a solicitor in drawing up an advance directive, which will definitely keep the cost down. Once your advance directive is signed, ensure that as many of the professionals and carers involved in looking after you as possible have a copy for their records.

This list of people may include your

- ✔ GP
- ✔ Consultant
- ✔ Specialist nurse
- ✔ Social worker
- ✔ Next of kin

And, of course, you can give your lawyer a copy for safe keeping too.

Looking into Lasting Power of Attorney

Another safeguard for people with dementia who lose capacity to make decisions is to appoint an attorney (or attorneys, if they want) to make those important decisions on their behalf.

Lasting power of attorney (LPA) is a document that sets out whom you (the 'donor') have instructed to be your attorney to make decisions on your behalf if you become unable to.

Two types of power of attorney exist:

- ✔ Health and welfare
- ✔ Property and financial affairs

You can choose to make one type or both.

Health and welfare lasting power of attorney

This document allows you to choose someone to make decisions for you concerning issues such as

- ✔ Your daily routine (what you eat and drink and what you wear)
- ✔ Medical care you receive, and treatments and investigations you do and don't want to receive (saying no to invasive tests and operations, for example)
- ✔ Moving from your own home into sheltered housing or a care home
- ✔ Life-sustaining treatment and resuscitation

Your attorney only makes these decisions on your behalf if you lose capacity. Certain decisions, however, can already be written into your advance directive; the attorney can't overrule decisions in your advance directive unless you've explicitly given him your permission to do so in the directive.

Property and financial affairs lasting power of attorney

This document allows you to choose one or more people to make decisions about money and property for you. The attorneys may take charge of

✔ Paying your bills

✔ Collecting benefits

✔ Selling your home

This type of lasting power of attorney can be used as soon as it's registered, with your permission, even if you still have full capacity yourself.

Taking a look at the benefits offered by lasting power of attorney

As any Boy Scout will tell you, it's best to be prepared. Setting up a lasting power of attorney document while you're in a good position to do so means you can cover all potential eventualities to your own satisfaction and you have the right people in place to look after you.

Lasting power of attorney also means that everyone who cares for you is aware at an early stage of your disease of your future plans and wishes. This is particularly important if you're on your own, or in a family where different members don't get along and may have their own, conflicting, ideas about what will be best for you.

Sorting out lasting power of attorney also makes sense from a financial point of view, because if you lose capacity to make decisions without a lasting power of attorney, your family will have to go through the Court of Protection to organise your affairs. This legal process is costly in both time and money and adds unnecessary stress at a time when life may already be difficult for all of you.

And finally, by putting your own attorney(s) in place, you avoid the risk of either a stranger or someone you know but don't trust making decisions for you.

Setting up lasting power of attorney

Just to make things a little less straightforward than necessary, slightly different processes are involved in setting up lasting power of attorney depending on whether you live in England and Wales, Scotland or Northern Ireland. Many of the details that follow for England and Wales are common throughout the UK, and I highlight those that are specific in the other two countries separately.

Choosing an attorney

You can choose one or more people as your attorney. Each person must be over 18 years of age and can be

- ✔ A relative
- ✔ A friend
- ✔ A professional (like a solicitor)
- ✔ Your husband, wife or partner

Choosing people you know and trust and who you believe will have your best interests at heart is a good idea. It's also not a bad idea to pick those who you know are good at looking after themselves and their own affairs. A great friend who's the life and soul of the party and great company down the pub, but who's up to his ears in debt and fond of a flutter at the races, may not be your best bet. By all means continue to enjoy such people's moral support and company, but don't give them control of your savings. And people who are bankrupt are specifically barred from being an attorney.

Dealing with the relevant paperwork

Unlike for advance directives, you need to fill in a specific form to apply for lasting power of attorney. This form is available from the Office of the Public Guardian, which is part of the Ministry of Justice. You can obtain the form by

- ✔ Filling it in online:

  www.gov.uk/lasting-power-of-attorney

- ✔ Downloading it from the government website and posting it back:

  www.gov.uk/government/publications/make-a-lasting-power-of-attorney

- ✔ Requesting that the form be sent to you, if technology isn't your thing and you prefer to use pen, paper and stamps, and then sending it back to:

  Office of the Public Guardian
  PO Box 16185
  Birmingham
  B2 2WH

  Tel: 0300 456 0300

As part of the information on the form you need to name a *certificate provider*. This person needs to have known you for at least two years or be professionally qualified to certify that he believes that you understand the lasting power of attorney process and its significance. This person will therefore often be your GP or solicitor.

Unfortunately, the paperwork component of the process doesn't end there. Once the form has been completed, it needs to be registered with the Office of the Public Guardian. You can apply to register yourself if you're the person appointing the attorneys (your title in this process is the *donor*), or the attorneys themselves can apply.

Before registering, you must notify up to five people who know you well (usually other friends and family members) about your application, and they have three weeks in which to raise objections to your choice of attorneys. This step is a final protective measure to ensure that your interests will be looked after as well as possible. If these five people are happy with your choice of attorneys, you can then fill out registration forms, again using the preceding contact details.

Once your lasting power of attorney is registered, a copy needs to be certified. If you still have capacity, you can do this yourself; if not, it can be registered by a solicitor or, somewhat bizarrely, a member of the stock exchange. (You can find details of the registration process on the website for the Office of the Public Guardian; www.justice.gov.uk/forms/opg.)

The whole process of setting up lasting power of attorney can take around eight weeks and costs a few hundred pounds, although means-tested discounts are available.

Considering regional variations

Slightly different processes apply in Scotland and Northern Ireland:

- **Scotland:** The initial stage of drafting a power of attorney is carried out by the *granter* (equivalent of donor) with the help of a solicitor, rather than by filling in an online form. A certificate of capacity must then be signed by either a solicitor or doctor, and finally you complete a registration form, which you obtained from the Scottish Office of the Public Guardian.

  www.publicguardian-scotland.gov.uk

- **Northern Ireland:** The term enduring power of attorney is used, and a solicitor draws up the document. This document is then registered with the High Court (Office of Care and Protection).

  www.nidirect.gov.uk/managing-your-affairs-and-enduring-power-of-attorney

The Court of Protection

According to the Ministry of Justice website, the role of the Court of Protection is to appoint deputies to act on behalf of and make decisions for people who are unable to make their own decisions about their personal health, finance or welfare.

The court is involved in cases whereby someone lacks capacity, as set out in the Mental Capacity Act 2005.

So, for example, the court will

✔ Make declarations about a person's capacity to make a decision, if the matter of this decision cannot be resolved informally.

✔ Make decisions in relation to providing, withdrawing or withholding medical treatment for a person who lacks capacity.

✔ Appoint a deputy to make ongoing decisions on behalf of a person who lacks capacity, in relation to either the person's personal welfare or property and financial affairs.

✔ Make decisions about lasting power of attorney, including whether the power is valid, objections to registration, and the scope and removal of attorney powers.

If the Court of Protection needs to be involved in any of these matters, forms must be filled in, hearings attended and a few hundred pounds paid in fees. Reaching a decision can take up to 16 weeks.

Setting up a lasting power of attorney as soon as possible is clearly the way to go!

Making Decisions about Resuscitation

While advance directives can stipulate which medical treatments you want withheld and when, including resuscitation, you can also specifically dictate your wishes regarding resuscitation in the event of you having a cardiac or respiratory arrest.

You need to have considered this very important scenario, because if an ambulance is called, without this piece of paper to hand the paramedics will be duty bound to begin resuscitation and transport you to hospital. You won't have a peaceful death with an ambulance crew jumping up and down on your chest and inserting needles into your veins, while zapping you with 360 joules of electricity to try to jump-start your ticker.

The paramedics will do all they can to bring you back, unless it's obvious to them that you're quite happy that when you're gone, you're gone.

Checking out the forms

Depending on where you live in the UK, you'll have to fill in a form specific to your NHS region that covers the same kinds of questions as elsewhere in the country. This form features the following information:

✔ Your name, address, date of birth and NHS number

✔ The name, address and contact number of your GP

It also has a section stating why carrying out cardiopulmonary resuscitation (CPR) is felt to be inappropriate in your case. This section commonly includes the following reasons, which the doctor must tick at least one of:

✔ Attempting CPR is unlikely to restart the patient's heart and breathing.

✔ No benefit will be gained from restarting the patient's heart and breathing.

✔ The expected benefit of the treatment is outweighed by the burdens and would not be in the best interests of the patient.

✔ Attempted resuscitation is against the competent patient's expressed wishes.

The doctor then has to either acknowledge that you have capacity to make this decision and that he's discussed it with you and your next of kin, or tick a box to say that you don't have capacity and that he's discussed it with the person who has lasting power of attorney.

Finally, a review date is included so that if things change the DNAR (do not attempt resuscitation) form can be rescinded.

'Do not resuscitate' does not mean 'do not treat'. If doctors or paramedics are given this form, they do all they can to ensure that your symptoms are managed as well as possible and that you're made comfortable. They won't take you to hospital and they won't start CPR if your heart stops or you stop breathing, but they will take very good care of you and do everything else necessary.

Telling the necessary people

If your GP's been through the form with you, he'll send a copy to everyone who needs to know. However, if you've filled it in in hospital or with a hospital or hospice doctor, it's best to get a copy for your GP so that he's also aware.

Your GP will let anyone and everyone who comes into contact with you clinically, especially in an emergency, know that a DNAR form is in place. This includes:

✔ The local ambulance service

✔ Your consultants in hospital

✔ The out-of-hours doctor service

Do not resusci-tat

In 2011 an 81-year-old woman from Norfolk took the unusual step of getting a tattoo, the first she'd ever had, in order that ambulance crews and doctors would be in absolutely no doubt about her resuscitation wishes should her heart or breathing stop.

Inked across her chest she had 'DO NOT RESUSCITATE', and, hedging her bets in case she was discovered lying face down, 'PTO' was tattooed across her back. Despite having an advance directive in place for 30 years, she told the national press at the time that the tattoo was to ensure that there was 'no excuse for not knowing what I think'.

As experts in medical ethics pointed out to the newspapers, despite her novel way of getting her message across, it would hold no weight legally, and without her advance directive paramedics would be duty bound to start CPR anyway.

All your friends and family should also be aware of the existence of this form and your wishes. In a panic situation, and without an understanding of what you want, dialling 999 will be second nature to them, and with no form to hand you'll be jumped on and zapped or taken to spend the night on a trolley in the accident and emergency department.

Dealing with Driving Regulations

In England, Wales and Scotland, the Driver and Vehicle Licensing Agency (DVLA) is the government agency that tries to ensure that everyone who sits behind the wheel of a motor vehicle is safe to drive and isn't going to pose a risk either to themselves or the lives of others. (The Driver and Vehicle Licensing Northern Ireland (DVLNI) does the same job in Northern Ireland.)

As dementia progresses, driving can become more dangerous. However, the decision to stop someone from driving shouldn't be taken lightly, because it will reduce his independence dramatically. A doctor thus generally takes a sensitive approach to the person with dementia while also making sure that other people's safety isn't compromised.

Acknowledging how dementia affects driving ability

A review paper published in the *British Medical Journal* in 2007 described crash data that showed that the risk of crashing if you're a driver with dementia doesn't increase until you've had the disease for about three years. *But*

because the severity of dementia can vary from person to person and because the risk of either you or someone else being injured or even killed is very real, your doctor will always tell you to contact the DVLA/DVLNI and will be duty-bound to do it himself if you don't. Failure to report a medical condition that can affect driving also leads to a fine of £1,000.

Informing the DVLA/DVLNI

When the relevant agency's been informed of your diagnosis, you'll be sent a questionnaire. It asks for information about your symptoms, the names of the doctors who're treating you and details of any medication you're taking. The agency also asks whether it can write to your GP and any hospital consultants to ask for a fuller medical report about your condition.

When the agency has all this information, it makes a decision about whether you're allowed to continue to drive. If it's still not sure, you may be asked to complete a formal driving assessment at one of the agency's test centres so that the relevant person can see for himself what your driving is like.

If you're able to continue driving, you'll be issued with a new driving licence, which will expire in approximately 12 months. After that period, you have to be reassessed. During that time, you need to ask friends and family members to keep an eye on the way you drive and to give you an early warning if things are getting worse.

You must also inform your insurance company of your diagnosis; if you don't, your insurance may not be valid, and you'll be at risk of prosecution.

Giving up your driving licence

If you've driven for many years and you're the only driver in your household, surrendering your licence for good can be quite upsetting. However, the last thing you want to do is put other drivers or pedestrians at unnecessary risk. And the money you'll save by not having to pay for petrol or any of the other running costs involved in owning a car can be spent on using other forms of transport such as buses and taxis.

Surrendering your licence doesn't have to mean the end of your independence, but it does mean that you'll be much safer, which has to be a price worth paying.

Part IV
Sorting Out Domiciliary and Longer-Term Care

The top five ways to ensure good-quality ongoing care

- **Don't jump the gun.** Ensure that the decision you make about the best type of care for the person you're looking after is driven by him and his level of need. If someone is still largely independent, a nursing home in which everyone else is bed-bound will drive him to distraction.

- **Arrange for an expert assessment.** If the person wants to stay in his own home for as long as possible, ask the local authority to carry out an assessment. If remaining at home is deemed safe and workable, the social worker and occupational therapist can advise you about adaptations, such as hand rails and raised toilet seats, and how much visiting care will be needed.

- **Visit selected care homes.** You wouldn't dream of buying a house without seeing it first and being able to ask the estate agent questions. The same is true when you're choosing a care home for someone you love. Visit the place to get a feel for it, and make sure you get the opportunity to talk to staff members *and* other residents and their families.

- **Check out funding.** Living in a care home doesn't come cheap. Prices vary depending on whether your loved one needs nursing or residential care and also in relation to geographic location. The value of the person's property and savings is used to calculate how much he needs to contribute, but it's not a certainty that he'll have to sell his house.

- **Plan for end-of-life care:** While the person still has capacity, it's a good idea to discuss his wishes regarding place of death and resuscitation under certain circumstances. If appropriate, help him write an advance directive indicating the treatments he would and would not like to undergo in the future if he's no longer able to speak for himself at that time.

Find tips on how to go about finding the best care home for someone with dementia at www.dummies.com/extras/dementia.

In this part . . .

- ✔ Consider the options for long-term care, looking at the pros and cons of each and choosing the right care home for the person you love.

- ✔ Help the person settle into the new home and make staff aware of the extent of the person's needs.

- ✔ Find out how to make a hospital admission as stress-free as possible for the person with dementia and staff.

- ✔ Look at how to experience a good death with dignified end-of-life care.

Chapter 16

Choosing Ongoing Care for Your Loved One

In This Chapter

▶ Making an informed and measured decision about suitable care

▶ Altering the person's home to meet her needs

▶ Picking the right care home

*F*or both people with early dementia and their carers, the subject of care can be a tricky one. The phrase 'don't you dare put me in a home' is one I commonly hear my elderly patients utter to their relatives; they think that if they have to move into one, they'll be out of sight and therefore out of mind.

For carers, making the decision to place someone in a care home invariably involves feelings of guilt. They don't want their loved one to be unhappy, but know that the increasingly complex needs of the person with dementia make it difficult to continue to provide care at home, especially because carers may well also have jobs to hold down and their own children to look after.

Clearly, the financial aspect also has to be considered. What care can the person with dementia afford; will she have to sell her house; and will there be any inheritance left for the family afterwards?

These are all important considerations, but the bottom line is that the needs of the person with dementia must come first. This chapter looks at the options – from care in the person's own home to full-time care in a nursing home – and the advantages and disadvantages of each.

Reaching a Realistic Decision

We obviously don't live in a perfect world, otherwise no one would develop dementia in the first place. You need to take this reality into consideration when looking at options for care. An option that suits the person with dementia 100 per cent is unlikely to exist, so you have to be prepared to find one that ticks most of your boxes, somewhere that's good enough. Otherwise the whole process can be extremely frustrating.

Being guided by how well someone is doing

This is by far the most important factor to think about when planning someone's future. When people with dementia are still living independently at home much of the time, but just need help with personal hygiene, cooking and shopping, then a nursing home, where people are confined to bed and need feeding, will drive them mad. They'll have no company and be bored. Likewise, if they're at the end stage of the disease and severely disabled by it, then a home carer popping in twice a day to wash their face and put a meal in front of them will be wholly inadequate too, especially if the person with dementia can no longer hold a knife and fork.

These scenarios may seem obvious, but in the panic engendered by a deteriorating situation, common sense can fly out of the window. You can avoid making the wrong decisions by asking some straightforward questions, such as:

- ✔ If the person needs help, how much does she need to make life simple for her?
- ✔ What are her main disabilities and what can be done to help work around them?
- ✔ Where do you need to draw the line to avoid stifling the independence she has left?
- ✔ Is she going downhill fast or is her deterioration slow and stepwise?

I'm sure you can think of your own questions, but they should all be aimed at solving the following equation, where X stands for level of care:

Current level of disability + X = Best quality of life possible

Considering whether symptoms are rapidly progressing

One other variable slightly complicates the equation in the preceding section and thus the decision that needs to be made. If someone has a rapidly progressive form of dementia, you have to factor it into the decision-making process to avoid having to move her from one setting to another in quick succession. Allowing a person to get settled somewhere and shortly afterwards putting her through the upheaval and undoubted confusion of another move is the worst thing possible for her. And it's equally frustrating (and financially costly) for families to think that the process is over and their loved one settled, only to have to go through it all again soon after.

You may be lucky and find some care homes locally that cater specifically for people with dementia and can alter levels of care as things progress. Another option is to keep someone at home as long as possible before making the move and then arranging care in a home with nursing support. Options vary throughout the country, which may prove limiting, but the process can certainly be made easier by planning ahead and speaking to all the professionals involved in the person's care to get their views on the matter. Speaking to care home managers about their own past experiences may also help you make up your mind.

Deciding whether existing help is sufficient

You don't have to rush into anything, and carrying out an initial mental stocktake of the support and input a person already receives and whether scope exists for it to be tweaked here and there if things start to go downhill is very useful. Possibly nothing needs doing at all yet.

In the midst of a seeming crisis it's very tempting to want to do _something_. And a knee-jerk reaction can lead to premature decisions that are either not yet necessary or, worse still, more disruptive than helpful. As Corporal Jones famously said in almost every episode of _Dad's Army_: 'Don't panic!' And if you're seeking advice about what to do, always speak to the person's GP or specialist nurse. She should have a good idea of the levels of help needed and the best people to carry out a thorough, objective assessment.

Making Alterations to the Existing Home

If the person with dementia is keen to stay put for a while and the family and medical staff agree that it's safe for her to do so, you need to consider how to make her life easier and safer in that setting. People often proudly refuse to let others into their homes to do chores, deliver food or help with toileting. But I always try to impress on them that the benefits hugely outweigh any potential embarrassment.

Having someone to help them do the things they're struggling with and spending far more time on than they need to gives people with dementia more time to do the things they enjoy. Plus, outside help frees family and friends, who are unlikely to be professional carers anyway, to spend more time doing enjoyable things with the person who has dementia rather than concentrating on laundry, vacuuming or scrubbing the toilets.

Asking whether a few simple changes are enough

In the early stages of dementia when cognitive and functional symptoms are likely to be the most prominent, the level of disability caused by the dementia may be quite low. However, forgetfulness and poor planning can affect people's ability to create a meal and produce a sensible shopping list. People may also begin to lose the desire to keep themselves and their homes clean. In this situation, particularly if the person still lives with a spouse or other family members, then what's needed may be quite simple. Of course, the level of care will need reassessing as time goes on, but the professional carers involved can help with that.

Looking at what's available

Being aware of the help that's potentially available can make the decision about where a person is safe to stay much clearer. If the person with dementia needs help with personal hygiene and cooking, for example, and no home care support or family members are available to help, the person may have to go into either sheltered accommodation or a residential care home anyway. If help is available, and thankfully that's most often the case, then staying at home with a greater degree of independence is definitely an option. A range of services can also be called upon even when the condition progresses.

Local authorities may offer the following types of help:

- **Shopping:** Home care staff help the person with dementia draw up a shopping list and then go to the supermarket.

- **Meals on wheels:** Run by volunteers, this is a very helpful and well-known service. It delivers hot meals or, if people want to choose when to have their lunch or tea, frozen meals that can be reheated in a microwave in their homes. The meals can be delivered daily or just a few times a week, and include a dessert. Meals on wheels also caters for specific dietary needs, providing vegetarian, soft, puréed, low-fat, gluten-free, diabetic, kosher and halal options.

✔ **Cleaning:** Home care staff can help people with dementia stay on top of domestic chores and housework, keeping their homes clean and safe. Doing so can include assistance with cleaning all the rooms in the house and dealing with refuse and recycling.

✔ **Washing and bathing:** As dementia progresses, people's co-ordination and ability to wash safely and frequently is often lost. Home carers can assist with bathing in the morning and before bed. Doing so may involve minor adaptions to the person's home, and an occupational therapist can help with this – see Chapter 11.

✔ **Mobility:** If people's mobility is affected by dementia, indoors or outside, a wheelchair can be a lifeline to ensure that they can still get some fresh air and that friends and relatives can still take them out and about.

Different types of chair are available: some fold up so that they fit in the car boot; others are electric and so can be operated by the person herself. Door frames can be adjusted to accommodate a wheelchair and a ramp put in to allow easy access.

✔ **Assistive technology:** Ranging from a 'Magi Plug' (www.magiplug.com) to avoid the bath overflowing and flooding the house, to installing Just Checking (www.justchecking.co.uk) movement sensors in each room to enable relatives to understand a person's routine. Finding that the person is more active at night may explain why she's sleeping during the day and missing out.

✔ **Home adaptations:** A large number of special aids and home adaptations are available to make life easier for people with increasing cognitive and physical difficulties. As the dementia goes on, previously straightforward tasks in the home become more of a struggle. Local authority or NHS occupational therapists assess a person's difficulties and provide suitable aids, including

- A walk-in shower with a seat

- A hoist for over the bath

- Raised toilet seats

- Hand rails throughout the house

- A stair lift

- Commodes

- Non-spill cups for drinking

- Large-faced clocks

Some funding may be available for these alterations and adaptations. However, they can also be purchased privately from specialist shops and on the Internet.

✔ **Sitting service:** Home care can provide day sitters to keep the person with dementia company while spouses and family carers go out.

✔ **Nursing care:** Nurses can come into the home to deal with dressings and wounds, and for catheter care and ulcer prevention.

Choosing a Care Home

Choosing a care home may be the next necessary step for one of two reasons:

✔ After reviewing current needs, it's been decided that the home is no longer a safe environment and more intensive input is needed.

✔ Someone has been cared for at home for a time, but the person's needs have changed as the condition has progressed and home care is no longer a viable option.

Whatever the reason, the next step involves yet more choices, because care homes vary in the level of care they provide. The three main options are

✔ **Sheltered housing:** Accommodation where a warden or, more often now, roaming staff offer help and support when needed.

✔ **Residential care:** A care home in which meals are provided and professional carers offer support, but no nursing provision is available on site.

✔ **Nursing home:** As the name suggests, a home staffed by qualified nurses who can provide high levels of care to the most disabled and incapacitated residents.

If the move is for the first reason and is the first residence away from the person's own home then all three options may be appropriate. If, however, people are moving from home after a period of care that's no longer suitable, sheltered accommodation is unlikely to offer anything more than they experienced at home, and the choice is thus between residential or nursing home care.

Differentiating Between Sheltered, Residential and Nursing Care Options

In order to help work out which may be best for the person's needs, I look at what each option has to offer in turn. I start at the lower end of the spectrum with sheltered accommodation and then work my way up the scale.

Sheltered accommodation/ extra-care housing

This type of housing can be provided by local authorities, charities or, more often these days, private companies. The accommodation may include houses, flats and bungalows all situated together on a single site. They're often purpose-built, low-maintenance, new developments. These buildings are self-contained and so have their own bedrooms, kitchens, bathrooms and living areas. They can accommodate either single people or couples, and are only available for people over retirement age.

Each house or flat has its own door key, giving the resident a sense of independence and privacy. However, a shared entrance may exist and also communal areas for social events, activities and informal conversation.

Some sheltered housing projects have a manager or warden on site during office hours. These people are available to answer queries and often pop in and review residents every day. If a resident needs medical help, the resident contacts the relevant person. Outside office hours, a 24-hour helpline is usually available so that staff from the housing organisation can be contacted around the clock. Not only do staff help with health and social issues but they also sort out practical problems like leaking taps and faulty electrics.

For people to be eligible for this type of accommodation, they must usually meet the following criteria:

- ✔ Their current home doesn't meet their needs.
- ✔ They have a medical or social need to move, such as an illness, a disability or a need to move to be nearer family.
- ✔ They're unable to buy a property themselves and need to rent instead.

If people are existing council or housing association tenants, they need to speak to their landlords about transferring to sheltered accommodation.

This type of accommodation may well suit people with early symptoms who can no longer cope with chores in a big house with a garden, but who think they'll find things far more manageable in a flat or bungalow. And the warden and out-of-hours emergency cover give families peace of mind.

Sheltered accommodation is especially suitable for couples in which one partner has dementia. The list of chores facing the healthy partner obviously reduces as a result of downsizing. Such accommodation is also available all over the country, so in the early stages people can move nearer to their relatives while not actually living with them, providing reassurance on both sides.

Residential homes

A residential home is the next step up in the care ladder. These homes cater for people who can still live independently to an extent but need help and prompting with many activities of daily living. A useful term to describe the support they provide is 'assisted living'.

Residential homes provide long-term, if not permanent, care for their residents, but can also sometimes offer short-term respite care. Respite care may cover convalescence after a period in hospital or provide carers with a much needed break to recharge their batteries.

These homes may be purpose built and run by the local authority or by chains of private companies. They're often large houses that have been converted by private owners to serve this function.

Residents benefit from

- ✔ Their own furnished or unfurnished room (so furniture and knick-knacks can be brought in to make it more homely)
- ✔ En suite or occasionally shared bathrooms
- ✔ Three meals per day served in a communal dining area
- ✔ Full housekeeping and laundry services
- ✔ Communal living areas for social events
- ✔ Around-the-clock carers to help with washing, mobility, dressing and even feeding if needed
- ✔ Staff who liaise with GPs and nurses during times of illness

Residential homes aim to provide a safe and friendly environment in which people's privacy and dignity are respected. They'll often provide enjoyable and stimulating activities and try to help meet a person's psychological, emotional and spiritual needs as well as minimise the effects of her physical difficulties.

Some homes do accommodate couples who can share a room, but most are for single people only. Obviously, people can go out – this type of home is certainly not a prison. However, doors are likely to be locked and visitors expected to sign in and out as a form of protection. And while locking doors may be considered as a deprivation of someone's human right to liberty, it's the least restrictive and proportionate measure that can be put in place to reduce the risk of harm.

Nursing homes

These homes are designed for people who need help with more complex needs that require the skills of trained nurses rather than simply professional carers. Lots are specifically set up to care for people with dementia. As with sheltered housing and residential homes, nursing homes can be owned and run by both local authorities and private organisations. Either way, they're regulated to make sure that the care they provide meets the standards of established best practice. They also provide both short- and long-term accommodation.

Nursing homes generally offer the following:

✔ Nurses on site providing 24-hour care

✔ Individual rooms with en suite facilities and some shared bathrooms with better access for hoists

✔ Doors that allow wheelchair access

✔ Meals and laundry and housekeeping services

✔ Support in terms of mobility, washing, dressing and feeding

✔ Communal areas for social events such as music therapy

✔ A garden

Finding the Right Place

I've already alluded to most of the things you need to consider when choosing the right type of care home. However, summarising the recommendations made by most of the relevant charities working in the area of dementia and elderly care won't hurt. The following advice is thus a round-up of the suggestions that such charities have made.

Decide on the care requirements

This decision should be made by the social workers, GPs and specialist nurses involved in the person's care, together with family members. The managers and staff of the different homes will also be happy to carry out a needs assessment to make sure that they can offer the person appropriate care. Together, this information will inform whether the person with dementia needs to be in sheltered housing, a residential home or a nursing home.

Pick the right location

Next is the decision about where to look for a suitable home. For example, would finding one in the local community so that the person can keep the same GP and stay close to friends, the local church or key relatives be best? Or should the move be to a different part of town so as to be near the person with power of attorney?

Draw up a shortlist

Once the type of care and location have been decided, you need to find homes that may fit the bill. Try searching online, via the social services department or perhaps follow the advice of the person's GP.

Read reviews of potential homes online and also consult reports on the websites of different care regulators around the UK.

See them for yourself

You wouldn't buy a new house or car without viewing it at least once. Clearly, when choosing somewhere for a loved one to live so that she can be safe and receive good care, a look is even more vital. Look at homes on your shortlist first and then narrow them down to one or two choices before suggesting that the person with dementia pays them a visit.

Try to get a feeling of what goes on there, the attitude of staff and the demeanour of other residents. Checking out the decor and general state of repair can also give you an idea about the staff's and owner's attitude to the place. It may even be possible to have a quiet word with families of existing residents if they're visiting when you are.

Compare prices

Once you're down to the final couple of choices, financial considerations may be the clincher (if they haven't already been earlier in the process). It may be that taking finances into account means making a compromise here and there, but sadly that's the way of the world these days.

Arrange a temporary stay

According to government guidelines, care homes, but not sheltered accommodation, should offer a temporary stay in a home before someone commits to moving in long term. A short stay allows the family and the person with dementia to get a better idea of whether the person will be happy there and whether it really is as good a home as it looks. Ask when you visit whether a short stay is possible.

Identifying Good Care

Choosing a care home for a parent or relative is as important as choosing a good school for a child. For a school, you probably consider small class sizes, a good Ofsted report, excellence in exam results and top sporting facilities, and choose one that ticks most or all of those boxes. Looking for schools is something many people are used to doing, but looking for care homes is often virgin territory. The NHS website (www.nhs.uk) lists the following examples of what constitutes good care in a nursing or residential home:

- ✔ The home offers new residents and their families or carers a guide (in a variety of accessible formats) describing what they can expect while they're living there. Ideally, residents of the home have helped to produce the guide.

- ✔ The majority of staff have worked there for a long time; they know the residents well and are friendly, supportive and respectful.

- ✔ The home involves residents, carers and their families in decision making, perhaps through regular meetings with staff.

- ✔ The home supports residents in doing things for themselves and maximising their independence, including keeping contact with the outside community.

- ✔ The home offers a choice of tasty and nutritious food, which residents may have helped to prepare.

- ✔ The home takes into account the needs and wishes of all residents, and provides a variety of leisure and social activities.

- ✔ The home offers a clean, bright and hygienic environment that's been adapted appropriately for residents, with single bedrooms available that residents can personalise.

- ✔ Staff respect residents' privacy and knock before they enter someone's room.

✔ Staff are well trained – for example, nurses who specialise in dementia care.

✔ Staff respect residents' modesty and make sure that they look respectable while also recognising that residents have a choice in what they wear.

✔ The home is accredited in end-of-life care.

Not all good homes observe all these things; those that do most seem right when you visit. Such homes that come in at the right price are definitely worth considering. The final step before making a decision is sussing out the home's reputation.

Checking the Home's Reputation

Like schools, GP surgeries and hospitals, care homes in the UK are regularly assessed by government inspectors to ensure that they reach appropriate legal standards. Each country in the UK uses a different regulator, but all provide similar reports that you can refer to when checking a potential care home's suitability for a relative.

England

In England, the organisation responsible for care home regulation is the Care Quality Commission (CQC). It regulates care homes by

✔ Carrying out announced and unannounced inspections

✔ Using inspectors from health and social care backgrounds, together with patients and carers, under the leadership of an experienced CQC manager

✔ Assessing whether the homes it visits are safe, caring, responsive to people's needs and well run

✔ Speaking with people who live in the homes, as well as their carers and staff members

✔ Observing what goes on in the homes and interviewing the management teams

The CQC publishes the results on its website (www.cqc.org.uk).

What values are regulators looking for?

All UK care homes, whether residential or nursing, are expected to adopt a number of values to ensure their residents receive the best and safest care possible. It can be a relief for families and people with dementia to know that such high standards are expected of whichever home they live in, no matter the price they pay, the location and whether they're privately funding it or receiving funds from the NHS or local authority.

As an example, here's the list displayed on the website of the regulator in Northern Ireland (source: www.rqia.org.uk):

✔ **Dignity and respect:** The uniqueness and intrinsic value of individual residents is acknowledged and each person is treated with respect.

✔ **Independence:** Residents have as much control as possible over their lives whilst being protected against unreasonable risks.

✔ **Rights:** Residents' individual and human rights are safeguarded and actively promoted within the context of services delivered by the home.

✔ **Equality and diversity:** Residents are treated equally and their background and culture are valued and respected. The services provided by the home fit within a framework of equal opportunities and anti-discriminatory practice.

✔ **Choice:** Residents are offered, wherever possible, the opportunity to select independently from a range of options based on clear and accurate information.

✔ **Consent:** Residents have a legal right to determine what happens to them, and their informed, genuine and valid consent to the care and support they receive is essential.

✔ **Fulfilment:** Residents are enabled and supported to lead full and purposeful lives and realise their ability and potential.

✔ **Safety:** Residents feel as safe as is possible in all aspects of their care and life, and are free from exploitation, neglect and abuse.

✔ **Privacy:** Residents have the right to be left alone, undisturbed and free from unnecessary intrusion into their affairs and there is a balance between the consideration of the individual's own and others' safety.

✔ **Confidentiality:** Residents know that information about them is managed appropriately and everyone involved in the home respects confidential matters.

Wales

In Wales, the Care and Social Services Inspectorate (CSSIW) regulates and inspects care homes. The process it uses is similar to that of the CQC in England, although the CSSIW carries out more unannounced inspections. The CSSIW publishes reports on its website (www.cssiw.org.uk).

Scotland

North of the border the regulatory body is the Care Inspectorate. It too carries out inspections of homes and posts reports on its website (www.careinspectorate.com).

Northern Ireland

Finally, in Northern Ireland the regulatory body is the Regulation and Quality Improvement Authority. Again, you can find reports on its website (www.rqia.org.uk).

Chapter 17

Receiving Assistance from the State

- -

In This Chapter

▶ Looking at how care homes are funded

▶ Applying for funding for yourself or a relative

▶ Distinguishing between facts and myths about who pays for what

- -

*I*f you've already flicked through previous chapters in this book, I may seem to be stating the obvious, but caring for someone with dementia is not a cheap business. The more disabling the condition is, the more extensive the care the person needs, and the costlier it obviously becomes when it has to be provided by someone else. When someone needs 24-hour support in order to carry out the normal activities of daily living, and when this care must be provided in a residential setting and therefore full board and lodgings must also be paid for, the price is considerable.

But it's not all bad news. Depending on circumstances, financial support to help meet these costs may be available. In this chapter I look at the possible sources of such funds and the ways in which they can be obtained. I also cover the options available to those who have significant savings, who unfortunately aren't entitled to financial support.

Looking at Who Pays for Care

The answer to 'Who pays?' may seem pretty straightforward: the family or the state. Unfortunately, the situation isn't quite as clear cut. First, state funding can derive from both the National Health Service (NHS) and local-authority social-services department. And second, even those whose financial circumstances mean that they're required to pay a considerable amount towards their own care may also be entitled to some top-up support from the state.

To get a better idea of what might be needed and why, I first look at how care homes are funded.

Funding covers care homes anywhere in the country, not just those situated locally.

Checking out how care homes are funded

Care homes are run by a variety of different organisations. In general, the homes are likely to be

- ✔ Privately owned by individuals or families
- ✔ Privately owned by large companies that have care homes across the country
- ✔ Run by local authorities (that is, by town or city councils)
- ✔ Run by charities with an interest in the elderly or in people with dementia, or by other voluntary organisations such as churches

The funding sources for each of these are clearly different. Privately owned homes are sustained by profits they make from charging residents and their families; local authority homes receive funds from local taxes via council budgets; and charities depend to some extent on donations from their supporters.

The amount of money needed to keep these homes operating depends on a number of different factors, such as the

- ✔ Size of the home and the number of bedrooms and facilities it offers
- ✔ Level of care provided: whether residential or full-on nursing
- ✔ Location of the home

Rents, mortgages, utility costs, council taxes and the price of groceries vary across the UK. Homes in London and the South East of England therefore have higher running costs (and therefore charge higher fees) than those in Scotland and the North East of England.

Taking all these variables into consideration, at the time of writing (in 2013/14) residential care costs an average £28,500 per year, and nursing home care £37,500 per year. Bearing in mind the North–South divide, weekly costs are in the region of

- ✔ **Residential care:** £489 in Yorkshire and Humberside; £641 in the South East
- ✔ **Nursing home care:** £603 in Wales; £874 in the South East

All other regions in the UK fall in-between these figures. These figures are just averages, however, and individual homes may well be cheaper or considerably more expensive.

Knowing what funds are available

With these sorts of sums in mind, you can easily see how, for most people, paying for residential care can break the bank. Unless you're fortunate enough to have extremely deep pockets or a winning National Lottery ticket, you need to check whether you can get funding to help with these charges.

Local authority funds

Local authority funding is the financial support that most people are aware of. Applicants are subject to a financial assessment, or means test. Clearly, the more savings someone has, the less likely he is to be awarded funding. However, on the flip side, the less money someone has, the more likely he is to receive financial assistance. And those somewhere in the middle may be able to access some support to top up their own finances.

Each local authority places an upper limit on the funds that people in need can receive, which obviously affects the sort of residential or nursing home care they can afford. As a result, for example, the person with dementia may have to live in a care home in a cheaper part of town or in a different area entirely. Thus, while the funds ensure that people are cared for at the level they require, it doesn't mean that they'll necessarily be able to live in a care home resembling the Ritz (unless they want to pay the extra cost themselves). They may have to make do with somewhere smaller or more homely, which may actually be no bad thing.

People who must meet the cost of their own care may still be able to qualify to receive one or more of the various benefits I cover in Chapter 14. They can then use these benefits to contribute towards care home fees, to take some of the pressure off their otherwise rapidly diminishing savings.

In the case of those receiving full local authority funding and state benefits, these will be taken in payment towards care home costs. A small amount will remain as a form of 'pocket money', however, so that the person still has some cash of his own.

NHS financial support

This source of financial support is perhaps less well known. And it's a well-kept government secret for good reason: it's not means tested and it's free.

NHS Continuing Healthcare is provided solely by the NHS and is available to people who have ongoing health needs outside hospital. It thus includes people being cared for in their own homes, as well as those needing residential or nursing care. This money can be used to pay for both health and social needs, so in a care home setting will completely cover board and lodging.

The funding is available to anyone over the age of 18 who has a significant primary health need. This means that any condition may qualify someone to receive NHS Continuing Healthcare, but he must first undergo an assessment to ensure that his condition merits the payment. Assessors examine the following four areas when assessing someone's suitability:

- **Nature:** The effects the condition has on him and his resulting care needs. Clearly, in dementia, the range of symptoms and level of disability they cause can be extensive.

- **Complexity:** Some conditions are obviously more straightforward to manage than others. Assessors look at the way in which someone's different needs present themselves and the type and level of skill required of carers to deal with the needs appropriately. In dementia, the person may have physical symptoms such as unsteadiness or incontinence, and psychological and behavioural issues.

- **Intensity:** This is a measure of the severity of the individual's condition and thus the ongoing level of support needed. In dementia, which is progressive, the person needs long-term care that will become more intense over time.

- **Unpredictability:** This considers not only the challenge that the person's condition poses for carers but also the risks to the person's health if carers fail to adapt to such challenges quickly and effectively.

To start the process of assessing need, a social or healthcare professional completes a checklist. If the checklist suggests that the person may be eligible for funding, the professional then contacts the local clinical commissioning group (CCG), which is responsible for NHS funding.

The CCG sets up a multi-disciplinary meeting to carry out a more detailed assessment of the four areas described in the preceding list, involving those professionals who are currently involved in the person's care, such as community nurses, social workers, GPs and physiotherapists.

If the person fits the criteria for receiving NHS Continuing Care, the multi-disciplinary team makes a recommendation to the CCG and hopefully funding is approved.

If the CCG decides that the person doesn't meet the criteria for NHS Continuing Care, the person or his family can appeal.

Even if funding is provided, however, the situation will be reviewed after three months and annually thereafter to assess ongoing eligibility. Being accepted for funding can involve a long slog, but it's ultimately worth it.

If someone is ineligible for Continuing Care funding, he may still be able to claim NHS-funded nursing care, money paid by the NHS to a nursing home to cover the cost of his care. Obviously, an assessment is necessary, but if someone's already been subject to a multi-disciplinary meeting, he won't need a further assessment. The only criteria that need to be met are that the person

✔ Has been assessed and requires the care of a registered nurse

✔ Is not eligible for NHS Continuing Care

Again, the decision will be subject to ongoing review, but in the case of someone with dementia, once he needs nursing care, he's sadly not going to get better.

Section 117 aftercare

Section 117 aftercare is free health and social care funding that is provided for people who have had a compulsory admission to hospital under the mental health act. These services can include help with accommodation, day care and recreational activities.

Calculating entitlement to funds

A *means test* is a tool to work out whether a person's entitled to local authority funding towards residential care, and if so, how much. As you can imagine, the powers that be won't part with their cash easily and they'll want to go over your finances with a fine-toothed comb.

The local authority looks at the following information:

✔ Bank and building society accounts

✔ Premium bonds and national savings

✔ Stocks, shares and investments

✔ Income from pensions (personal, state and occupational)

✔ Property and land deeds

It doesn't look at

✔ War widow's payments

✔ Payments for the mobility component of the Disability Living Allowance

> ✔ Income from a spouse's pensions
>
> ✔ Property that continues to be occupied by a partner or dependent

For calculation purposes, any funds held in joint accounts are divided in half to calculate the relevant share. Once the local authority has calculated the amount, the funds will be allocated. You can ask the local authority to send details of how it worked out the funding.

Examining Self-Funding

So, if you've had no luck applying for local authority funding for residential home care, what happens next? How do you pay for the necessary care, and where do the funds come from? Will the council raid your bank account or sell the roof from over your head?

Many people fear that in taking care of someone in need, they're kissing good-bye to the property and savings they've worked for all their lives; they worry they'll leave nothing to pass on to the next generation. In this next section I take a look at the facts.

Considering whether you'll have to sell your house

An Englishman's home is his castle (as is that of a Scottish, Welsh or Northern Irish man). Selling your home is a very big deal. Working out whether it will be necessary, however, isn't straightforward and depends on a number of different factors. You may have to sell the house of the person going into care, but you may not.

Below are a few specifics that will hopefully make things clearer. The house will not have to be sold (and will, in official parlance, be 'disregarded') if the house is occupied by

> ✔ The current partner of the person going into care
>
> ✔ An older relative over the age of 60 or a younger adult who is considered incapacitated
>
> ✔ The person's ex-partner who is also a lone parent
>
> ✔ Someone under the age of 18 who is still the responsibility of the person going into care

✔ Someone under the age of 60 who's been looking after the person going into care (this point is completely at the discretion of the local authority)

In a few other instances, you can avoid selling up immediately, even if the criteria above cannot be met:

✔ If someone who doesn't fit the categories in the preceding list lives in the house, you can delay selling until he moves out, at which point you can pay the income from the sale back to the local authority.

✔ You can avoid selling altogether by renting the house out and using the income to pay the care home bill.

✔ Even if you do eventually have to sell the house to meet the costs of residential care, a period of 12 weeks' grace may be given during which the local authority will foot the bill while the house is put on the market and sold.

A local council, like an elephant, never forgets. If the house isn't sold within a set time, the council will still recoup the money you owe it when the house is sold.

Likewise, don't assume that you'll get away with paying fees by selling a house and giving the money to relatives as an inheritance before you go into a residential home. The local authority will ask about this sort of sale and can insist that you use the assets raised to pay for care.

Identifying which pensions and savings will be used

To repeat, you can be expected to dip into the following pensions and savings to pay for a place in a care home:

✔ Personal, state and occupational pensions

✔ Bank and building society accounts

✔ Premium bonds or national savings

✔ Stocks, shares and investments

The good news is that once your savings and so on are used up and you meet local authority funding criteria, the local authority will reassess your financial situation and may bear the cost of residential care.

Recognising whether the family will be stuck with a bill

Not so long ago, before 2009 to be precise, local authorities could make spouses or civil partners contribute to their loved ones' care home costs. Since then the rules have changed so that the only person liable for the fees is the person going into care.

If someone is entirely self-funding, however, the family will have to settle any unpaid fees from his estate. This payment is unlikely to be huge, though.

Similarities and differences in care home funding across the UK

Most of the details about funding and assessment in this chapter apply to England and Wales. The situation may be different in Scotland and Northern Ireland – although it by no means always is – because of the way in which power to dictate health and social care policy is devolved from the national government in Westminster to their respective governments in Edinburgh and Belfast.

For example, in Scotland:

✔ Everyone contributes to their care home fees, the amount varying according to the level of each person's capital and savings and the cost of the home itself.

✔ Rules about which savings and when a house needs to be sold are similar to those for England and Wales.

✔ People moving into a care home will need to have a new assessment of their care needs even if they had one while living in their own homes.

✔ The details concerning NHS Continuing Care are the same as those applied to England and Wales.

And in Northern Ireland:

✔ Like in Scotland, everyone's expected to contribute, and the amount varies according to income and savings.

✔ The rules about which savings are used and when a house must be sold are the same as those applied across the UK.

✔ NHS Continuing Care may cover nursing fees.

For more specific details of residential and nursing home funding in the different regions of the UK, head to the following web pages:

England: www.nhs.uk/Carers Direct/social-care/Pages/ funding-your-care.aspx

Wales: http://wales.gov.uk/ topics/health/socialcare/ care/?lang=en

Scotland: www.scotland.gov. uk/Topics/Health/Support- Social-Care/Financial-Help/ Charging-Residential-Care

Northern Ireland: www.nidirect. gov.uk/residential-care-and- nursing-homes

Chapter 18

Helping the Care Home

- -

In This Chapter

▶ Introducing someone to care home staff

▶ Looking at the benefits of visiting regularly

▶ Getting involved in aspects of care

▶ Knowing what to do if things go wrong

- -

*W*hen you've decided on the best care home to look after your loved one, it's time to help settle her in. The more information you can give the new carers, the better able they are to make the person with dementia feel at home as quickly as possible. The person will no doubt feel unsettled by having to move out of either her own home, which she may have shared with a spouse, or your home if she's been with you temporarily. Either way, her surroundings would have been familiar, along with the faces of those looking after her, even if she didn't always remember who they were. Now she's in an unfamiliar place, surrounded by strangers.

And even more disconcerting, other people are sharing the place with her: new people to get to know and with whom to share the TV, dining table and toilet facilities. In a care home, people are no longer able to completely please themselves, and even if they do have their own rooms to escape to, they'll have to get used to the art of communal living.

Getting the Home Care Staff to Know Your Loved One

Helping the manager and staff of the home to get as clear a picture of the new person as soon as they can is my first tip. Doing so involves informing them about the person's history and family background, diagnosis, treatment needs, likes and dislikes, and anything else you think they could do with knowing to smooth things all around.

The carers in the home are likely to complete a file on each resident containing this sort of information. And no doubt they'll ask a standard set of questions of everyone who moves in. But no harm exists in you anticipating these standard questions by drawing up a list of things you want to tell them yourself and actually going further by giving them details of things they may not even think to ask.

Providing important biographical details

The amount of information provided here needs to be somewhere between the sort of things the person may have told a stranger at a dinner party about herself and a print-out of her full CV. You don't want to leave the staff with any lingering question marks about the person, but neither do they need to be bored to death by details of how she loved annual trips to Cleethorpes to top up her thimble collection in the local gift shops.

Background and family

'No man is an island, entire of itself,' wrote John Donne. We all have connections with other people who are important to us, and we all have a life story that goes some way to explaining how we got to where we are today. To be able to understand us, others thus need to know a bit about where we've come from. Carers find it useful to have at least the following pieces of information about their new resident:

✔ **What she likes to be called:** This detail may seem obvious, but not all Terrences like to be known as Terry, and I have a patient named Irene who's always been called Marge. She gets really cheesed off when I forget and call her from the waiting room using the wrong name.

✔ **Her age, date of birth and where she was born:** Remembering someone's birthday is a vital way to show that you care, and the staff in the home will want to make a fuss of a person on her birthday each year to make her feel special and make sure she knows that her carers have a genuine interest in her.

✔ **Where she's moved from and why:** Numerous reasons may account for the person moving into the care home, such as an inability to cope in her own home, her needs becoming more complex so she can no longer live with a family carer or maybe being transferred directly from hospital after a period of illness that's caused a general deterioration. Knowing the reason for the move helps the staff to ease the transition, and if your loved one has moved in because you were struggling to look after her, staff can support you in your decision.

✔ **Whether she's been married, and if so, whether her spouse is still alive:** An awareness of wedding anniversaries and the date partners died helps the home anticipate days when people may be sad and withdrawn or perhaps a bit tetchy. The person may, of course, also have a special friend who visits her. Maybe she's homosexual, which the staff need to know to prevent any unintentionally awkward discussions.

✔ **Who's who in the family:** Identify who may visit, highlighting the person who has power of attorney and any 'tricky' relationships that exist within the family.

✔ **Previous occupation and military service, if applicable:** Some dates may trigger specific emotions and memories, as may seeing TV footage of battles or old soldiers. Maybe the person would like to be taken to a remembrance service too, especially if she's always attended in the past.

✔ **The names and species of past and present pets:** Possibly she's had to leave loved pets behind or will talk about deceased pets as though they're still alive.

✔ **Drinking and smoking habits:** Just because someone's older and has dementia doesn't mean that she's immune to having an interesting relationship with alcohol. This may manifest itself in regular swigs from a hip flask or the emergence of a wild or amorous side after a glass of sherry at Christmas. Either way, if the staff know about the possibility of problems with alcohol, they can anticipate and deal with them.

Likewise, if the person smokes and smoking isn't allowed indoors, she may need regular trips outside for a puff to avoid withdrawal symptoms and associated irritability.

Likes and dislikes

While homes aren't able to cater for absolutely every one of their residents' dietary likes and dislikes, it certainly helps them to know if a certain food makes a person feel sick and what she particularly enjoys for a special occasion. Likewise, if they know about a person's interests they can plan trips and activities that may at least tickle most people's fancies.

Do tell the home about the person with dementia's

✔ **Favourite food and drink:** Supplement this information with details of things she absolutely cannot bear and any allergies or special dietary requirements she has. Homes can cater for special diets, such as those for people with coeliac disease and diabetes, and they also provide meals suitable for people of different religious faiths.

✔ **Hobbies she's enjoyed or shown a passing interest in:** Maybe someone has always liked painting or knitting; maybe you think she'd enjoy gardening and may develop an interest in that. Many homes have gardens that residents are free to potter about in.

✔ **Musical tastes and dislikes:** If someone fails to show up to see a jazz band playing in the home, the staff will find it helpful to know that the person isn't ill or being odd or moody, but simply can't stand that type of music.

✔ **TV programmes and films she enjoys watching and those she doesn't:** Such information may help explain why someone starts shouting when the football comes on or someone else flicks the channel over to watch *EastEnders*.

✔ **Sleeping habits:** Is she an early bird or night owl, and does she have a tendency to wander?

✔ **Things that always make her bad-tempered or jolly:** Tell staff the best way to cheer a person up if she's a bit on the grumpy side.

✔ **Her religious beliefs, if any:** Inform staff if someone is a member of a local church, mosque or synagogue, for example, together with the name of the church leader. It may be possible for a member of the congregation to collect the person each week. If that's the case, the staff will appreciate advance notice so that they can get the person ready in time.

Covering medical details

Although a GP will always be sent the full medical notes of a new patient, the situation isn't the same for a care home, even if it's a nursing home. The carers must thus rely on relatives to bring them up to speed with the most relevant parts of the new resident's medical history.

Ongoing medical conditions

The person's GP may provide a printed-out summary of the person's current medical condition for you to give to the home. If the GP doesn't, however, the home will want to know if the person has

✔ Breathing conditions such as asthma, bronchiectasis or chronic obstructive pulmonary disease (COPD)

✔ Diabetes

✔ Heart disease, including angina, high blood pressure, heart failure or a history of actual heart attacks

✔ A history of any neurological conditions such as Parkinson's disease, epilepsy, headaches or migraines, strokes or mini strokes

✔ Arthritic joints, which affect mobility and may be very painful

✔ Mental health conditions (on top of their dementia) such as anxiety, depression or bipolar disorder

✔ A proneness to bowel troubles from simple indigestion and constipation through to stomach ulcers or inflammatory bowel diseases such as ulcerative colitis or Crohn's disease

✔ Skin conditions like eczema, dermatitis, psoriasis or a proneness to skin cancer or leg ulcers

✔ Impending investigations or major operations, or ongoing hospital follow-up appointments

✔ Visual or hearing difficulties

✔ Rare or unusual conditions that aren't covered by the preceding items in this list

Thankfully, most people don't suffer lots of simultaneous conditions, but giving the home details of any of these things can help the staff anticipate trouble and monitor the person for new or different symptoms, so they can involve the GP sooner rather than later.

Pills and prescriptions

If they're going to be dishing out pills and applying creams from the person's regular prescription list, the carers obviously need to know exactly what's on that list. They also need to understand which medicines are to be given daily regardless of symptoms and which are prescribed for use as and when a problem exists.

Inform the care home if the person with dementia is allergic to any medicines.

The GP surgery should be able to let you have a print-out detailing all the person's repeat prescriptions to give to the home. Possibly, the medicines are already delivered in a blister pack (see Chapter 11) and the arrangement can be transferred to the care home.

If the person is prone to recurrent infections, informing the home which antibiotics have been most effective in the past is a good idea. The person's own GP may know that detail, but an out-of-hours doctor will find it useful.

Identifying who's already involved in care

These details aren't so important if the person is in a care home in a totally new area, because her medical and social teams will probably change as a result of changing GP. But if the care home is close to where the person has been living and she's not changing doctors, give the care home the following information:

✔ The GP's name, to ensure continuity of care, along with the name of another GP at the practice whom the person may request to see if the first GP is unavailable

✔ The names of community matrons, community nurses for older people or district nurses, who may monitor chronic conditions or who visit to attend to ulcers or ongoing dressings

✔ The name and location of the person's dentist, podiatrist, optician, dietician, physiotherapist or speech and language therapist, if applicable

✔ The name of the hospital dementia specialist or memory nurse who's been keeping an eye on the person

✔ The name and contact details of the social worker who has co-ordinated the person's care

Do let the home know if any of these professionals are scheduled to visit, so that they can prepare the person in advance. Likewise, let the home know the dates of impending hospital trips too.

Visiting Regularly

Many people fear that when they're 'put in a home', their family and friends will neglect them and they'll be forgotten about. And I've actually heard relatives defend their lack of visits to elderly relatives by saying, 'Well, they don't know whether I've been in or not, so it doesn't matter how often I go.'

Well, the person in the home may well remember whether you've put in an appearance and be upset if you don't turn up for months. And even if she doesn't remember, surely she deserves better. Possibly, you're worn out from acting as the main carer and see the person's admission to a care home as the green light for some well-earned rest. And that's understandable. However, don't leave extended periods between visits, especially when the person is getting used to a new environment. Your visits may be just what she needs to help her settle in, and may give you peace of mind, knowing that she's well looked after and happy. Plus emotional memory may stay, so enjoying a visit may leave the individual feeling happy, even if she doesn't remember why. Remember, a person may not recall an event but she will remember how it made her feel.

Your visits can be ad hoc to fit in with your own schedule, but given the benefit of routine for people with dementia, visiting on set days is probably a good idea if you can manage it. Involving other members of the family is also beneficial, especially grandchildren, who are likely to bring a lot of pleasure to the person with dementia.

Tell the person's old friends where she's living and encourage them to visit too. Receiving old friends in this new environment will make it feel more like home. Maybe the friends will also be able to take the person out for a walk, or a coffee if she's still able to get in a car.

Care homes aren't scary places to visit, and other residents also value and benefit from seeing different people about the place, especially children. Neither are care homes intended to feel like prisons to their residents. Bring in familiar things from the person's old home, such as favourite books, family photos and other objects that may help her reminisce and also make the home feel like home.

Try to visit regularly and to make the person's life more interesting by taking her out on trips if she's up to it.

Taking Part in Care and Activities in the Home

Research suggests that good relationships play a vital role in improving the quality of life of people with dementia living in residential and nursing homes. Good relationships cover those with other residents and staff within the home and, just as importantly, with family and old friends. Even people with severe dementia have been shown to benefit.

When you visit the care home, don't just make a flying visit every time – try to hang around and participate. This level of engagement not only helps you get to know the staff of the home better, but also improves the mood and reduces the anxiety of the person you're visiting. Residents who've been surveyed also say that an engaged visit improves their feeling of hope.

In order not to get under the feet of staff, avoiding bath- and mealtimes at first is probably best. But as you get to know the carers in the home, you can ask whether you can go in at those times to be involved too. Think about participating in the following kinds of activities:

- ✔ Tea parties
- ✔ Visits from entertainers
- ✔ Trips out for the day
- ✔ Knitting or sewing groups
- ✔ Music therapy
- ✔ Exercise classes
- ✔ Meal-, bath- and bedtimes
- ✔ Palliative care at the end of life

Acting As an Advocate If Problems Occur

By visiting regularly and taking an active part in some of the home's activities, you send a clear message to the person with dementia that having gone into a home she's far from out of sight or out of mind.

You may also notice things that you're not happy with regarding the way your loved one is treated or the home is run. By visiting, you'll be more available for the person to tell you about issues that perhaps annoy or upset her too. British people are known for not wanting to make a fuss; they stiffen the upper lip and put up with it. But given some recent high-profile news reports of treatment of residents in UK care homes, you need to be vigilant.

Thankfully, these cases of mistreatment and neglect are rare, and regular inspections throughout the UK mean they're likely to become even less frequent. People who choose to run and work in residential and nursing homes are generally extremely patient, kind and caring individuals who do a very physically and emotionally demanding job to the best of their ability.

Vulnerable people with dementia need others to speak up for them. Little difficulties can become significant problems if people can't speak for themselves and nobody is looking out for them either.

Considering typical problems

Problems can be of a physical, emotional, psychological and even a structural nature, affecting both the person in the home and the state of the building she's living in.

Some particular areas for concern are

- ✔ **Level of personal care:** Are people in clean clothes, are they changed quickly if they have accidents or spillages, and do they have regular washes, baths and showers?

- ✔ **Quality and quantity of food:** Does everyone get their fair share at mealtimes, are decent portions offered, do the meals vary, are residents helped to the dining table if needed, is food cut up if necessary and is food taken to residents' rooms if they're feeling ill or out of sorts? And are they assisted to eat if necessary?

- ✔ **Cleanliness:** Are bathrooms, toilets and commodes thoroughly cleaned? Does the home smell of urine?

- ✔ **Staff professionalism:** Do staff behave appropriately and professionally at all times, or are they rude to residents or even neglectful? And do they talk over or about residents without acknowledging them?

- ✔ **Resident behaviour:** Do people seem happy and relaxed or are they stressed, anxious and uncomfortable in their surroundings?

If you find yourself providing a few negative responses to these questions, you need to take up the issues with someone in authority to make sure they're sorted out swiftly and appropriately.

Making a complaint

By law, all care homes must have a written complaints policy; you can ask for a copy of it when your loved one moves in. The policy will state to whom you should address your complaint, the type of response you can expect and how promptly.

Speaking to a manager or carer at the home informally at first is probably best. A straight conversation is often the simplest (and least stressful) way to deal with things. But if your concerns aren't dealt with to your satisfaction, a formal complaint is necessary.

You can express your complaint in writing (in a letter or email) or verbally (over the phone or in person). If you lodge your complaint verbally, make a written note of what's said.

Escalating the complaint

If you make a complaint and it's rejected out of hand, brushed aside or not dealt with to your satisfaction by the care home staff and management, the complaints procedure has to move up a gear. If you live in England, you can contact the Local Government Ombudsman (LGO). Complaints can be made to the LGO about care provided in the person's home and in homes managed by either private owners or the local authority. The LGO looks at complaints relating to

- ✔ Poor-quality care
- ✔ Fees and funding
- ✔ Poor complaint handling
- ✔ Unsatisfactory care needs assessment
- ✔ Safety and safeguarding

You can contact the LGO to log a complaint at any point in the 12 months following the incident, although doing so as soon as possible is best while the facts are fresh in your mind. The LGO is impartial and doesn't take sides but will investigate the facts to see whether the complaint should be upheld and what action should be taken to resolve the matter.

You can contact your local LGO via the LGO website (www.lgo.org.uk) or contact it by phone on 0300 061 0614.

If you live in Wales, Scotland or Northern Ireland, you have recourse to similar sorts of help from the three different organisations operating in those countries:

- ✔ **Wales:** Care and Social Service Inspectorate Wales at www.cssiw.org.uk and on 0300 7900 126
- ✔ **Scotland:** Care Inspectorate at www.careinspectorate.com and on 0845 600 9527
- ✔ **Northern Ireland:** Northern Ireland Ombudsman at www.ni-ombudsman.org.uk and on 02890 233821

Of course, if you're really unhappy about the care someone has received, you can seek advice from a solicitor, but dealing with the care home directly or involving an ombudsman are both more likely to resolve the situation to the benefit of both your loved one and other residents who may have similar concerns. The services of the LGO are free, and you can therefore avoid the cost of pursuing legal action.

Sources of support when making a complaint

Complaining isn't something (most) people do lightly, and the process can be difficult to work out and very stressful. The following organisations provide advice and support on navigating complaints processes:

✔ NHS Complaints Advocacy Service

nhscomplaintsadvocacy.org

Telephone: 0300 330 5454

The organisation offers free advice about the procedure for complaining about any NHS-funded service.

✔ Patient Advice and Liaison Services (PALS)

www.nhs.uk/service-search/ patient-advice-and-liaison- services-(pals)/location search/363

PALS is a national service supporting patients who have concerns about local NHS services, and their families. It has no central website, but your local PALS can be found via the link to NHS Direct above.

✔ The Relatives and Residents Association

www.relres.org

Telephone: 0207 359 81367

This association provides a helpline to support individuals and their families who have concerns about the care being received in residential and nursing homes.

✔ Citizens Advice

www.citizensadvice.org.uk

This service provides free and confidential advice to people on any aspect of their rights and responsibilities.

Chapter 19

Knowing What to Do If the Person with Dementia Goes into Hospital

. . . .

In This Chapter

▶ Ensuring communication is a two-way process

▶ Identifying the staff

▶ Providing stuff from home

▶ Taking time to visit

▶ Offering assistance during lunch and dinner

. . . .

Going into hospital can be a nerve-wracking experience at the best of times. I remember my first and, thankfully so far, only admission to hospital as if it was yesterday. And it wasn't yesterday: it was December 1973, and I was 6 years old. I can still bring to mind the regimented routine of the place and being alone at night, because in the less enlightened 1970s parents weren't allowed to stay with their children. What stuck out most, however, was the feeling of being a complete outsider in a strange world.

Hospitals are unnerving, strange and scary places for all of us, particularly if they're associated in our minds with trauma or the loss of a loved one. So imagine how much more scary they can be for people with dementia, who may not recognise where they are or the people around them, or understand what's happening to them and why.

Some hospitals do have mental-health liaison teams who will help general ward staff by assisting them when people with dementia are admitted into one of their beds. But this is not always the case. Either way this chapter has suggestions for ways in which you as a carer or family member can help someone with dementia to acclimatise to hospital life.

Communicating with Staff

If the admission is planned, the person with dementia will probably go straight to the hospital ward on which he's staying. If he experiences an unplanned emergency admission, however, as the result of a chest infection, heart attack or stroke, then admission may not be so smooth.

First stop may well be the accident and emergency (A&E) department. The person with dementia can spend an hour or two getting to know the staff there before being found a bed on one of the wards. Unfortunately, it's not unheard of for a patient to be moved again, from a short-stay admissions ward to a longer-stay ward somewhere else in the hospital.

Imagine how unsettling this process is for a patient with dementia. Regardless of how admission takes place, helping the person to get to know each new set of staff (and bear in mind that they'll change shifts several times in each 24-hour period too) is vital. You also need to make sure that the staff know and understand the person they're looking after.

Giving the staff some background history

Doctors, nurses and everyone else on the ward who comes into contact with patients will try to treat them as individuals and not according to their pathology – 'the spleen in bed four'. Unfortunately, we're all human, and on a busy ward, with frequent staff and patient changes over the course of the day, that ideal situation doesn't always match reality.

A danger also exists that when staff members hear the word 'dementia' they'll jump to conclusions about the condition. This issue can be a particular problem on wards unused to treating people with dementia, such as surgical wards, rather than on those geared up for elderly care problems or mental health difficulties.

To avoid misunderstandings, give the staff as much information as you can about the patient, as early on in the admissions process as possible. Useful information includes

✔ **The fact that the person has dementia and which type:** This may seem a bit obvious, but if admission has occurred via A&E, the staff may not have a full set of notes. An awareness of the type of dementia is also important to help try to predict particular difficulties the person may have. People deserve bespoke rather than standard, one-size-fits-all treatment.

✔ **The name the person likes to be called by:** Staff often don't know whether to be formal and go for 'Mrs Brown' or informal and use 'Celia'. Some patients feel patronised by over-familiarity while others find being addressed by their title and surname impersonal and uncaring. Problems may also be caused if someone's first name is 'Richard' but he's always been known as 'Keith' (it happens). Unless staff are told otherwise, obviously they'll always use the name on the medical records.

✔ **Details of other illnesses:** Tell staff about other medical conditions such as arthritis or emphysema, their effects and how best to minimise the symptoms. If a patient is in hospital with a urine infection, it may not cross the minds of staff to provide painkillers for arthritis in the patient's knee unless told to do so.

✔ **An explanation of daily self-care routines:** This covers those activities that need prompting and those the person will need help with. Activities include everything from brushing teeth to using a toilet. Shaving is an important one. A beard or moustache can be part of the person's identity, with upsetting consequences for the individual and family if it's removed; whereas if Dad has not been self-caring recently, a good, thorough shave can add to his feeling of wellbeing.

✔ **Any special dietary requirements or intolerances:** Such details don't simply cover the big things like an allergy to seafood or being a lifelong vegan; it's also helpful for staff to know if someone can't stand liver or hates custard on puddings. Particularly point out foods the person physically can't chew or has trouble swallowing. Refusal to eat may otherwise be seen as a behavioural problem, or even lead to malnourishment while on the ward. My mother hates pasta; try to make her eat that every day in hospital and she'll fade away.

✔ **Social background:** These details cover names of pets and important family members whom the person is especially close to; what sort of place he lives in; whom he lives with or whether he's alone; and any recent dramatic life events such as a bereavement. These facts not only help staff put names to faces of visitors, but also help them understand if the person talks in the present tense about people and events from the past. Also let the staff know if your loved one is someone who likes his own company, never one to mix, or whether the isolation he may feel while in hospital will have a negative impact.

✔ **Religious or cultural practices:** Chaplains serving all faiths practise in hospitals, and arrangements can be made for a patient to attend services.

✔ **Details of who has power of attorney, any advance directives and the existence of a 'do not resuscitate' order:** Clearly, it will be very distressing for everyone concerned if a patient is resuscitated against his wishes. Make sure you provide up-to-date phone numbers so that staff can contact you in an emergency.

Providing details about the person's care

Alongside tips on how to make the place more familiar for someone with dementia, in order to minimise the possible distress of new surroundings, the staff will also appreciate knowing how best to ensure that established routines are observed as much as possible and how to minimise agitation if things go wrong. Give staff information on

- ✔ The best way to communicate; for example, slowly and precisely and covering one important issue at a time.
- ✔ Whether the patient needs help with eating and drinking or can manage alone if the food is cut up or always served with ketchup.
- ✔ What sort of behaviours to watch out for that may suggest pain or a need to go to the toilet, if the person isn't good at mentioning these things directly.
- ✔ Whether the person needs help with washing or dressing, and whether he prefers to be assisted by a man or a woman to avoid distress and embarrassment.
- ✔ Whether agitation can be settled or avoided by encouraging the person to be active and mobile around the ward or hospital. As a junior doctor, I often came across one of my own patients with dementia in different places around the hospital; she'd get bored of her own surroundings and go off for a wander.

Getting to Know the Ward Staff and Doctors

Communication always works best when it's a two-way process, so as well as providing staff with information about the person in their care and introducing yourself, take time to get to know them too. The hospital can help with this process, because each patient should have

- ✔ A named doctor who's in charge of overseeing his care
- ✔ A named nurse who's available to chat to relatives about what's happening during the patient's stay on the ward

The names of both these professionals should be displayed on each patient's bed so that everyone knows whom to turn to for information.

Who's who in hospital

Hospital is a strange world for most of us, populated by people in different uniforms with strange Latin-based job titles that definitely don't make sense in plain English. Here's a quick whizz through the different professionals you may encounter in the wards and departments and a guide to their ranks and pecking order.

Doctors

Hospitals are full of doctors of various grades and specialities. You'll encounter relatively junior doctors on the ward and more senior doctors in outpatient clinics and operating theatres. The grades (from lowest to highest) are the same for each speciality:

✔ **Foundation doctors:** These newly qualified doctors are the most junior members of the medical team; they stay at this grade for two years before moving on to training in a speciality of their choice.

✔ **Specialty registrars:** Doctors stay at this grade for six years while they undergo training and take exams in their chosen speciality. They gain more experience as they proceed through the grade and are correspondingly given more responsibility as they progress.

✔ **Consultants:** These doctors have completed all their training and are the named doctors for patients on the wards, with overall responsibility for their care. They have a team of junior doctors working with them. In England and Wales, consultant surgeons are addressed as 'mister', and all other consultants are referred to as 'doctor'. In Scotland and Northern Ireland, all consultants are called 'doctor'.

Many hospitals work with undergraduate medical students. The students spend time talking to and examining patients on the wards to help them learn about different diseases and treatments, and hopefully people too.

Nurses

As with doctors, so a hierarchy exists among nurses too:

✔ **Healthcare assistants:** These men and women work alongside nurses to provide all kinds of general care to patients, from washing and dressing to taking observations and even making the beds.

✔ **Staff nurses:** These people make up the majority of nursing staff you see on the ward; they're graduates in nursing and have extra training in the speciality they're working in.

✔ **Ward sister/charge nurse:** This is a management role and a nurse with either title will be responsible for the smooth running of each hospital ward.

Other professionals

You may come across the following staff members either when visiting the ward to see a patient or in their own hospital departments:

✔ **Dieticians:** These have expertise in advising patients on all aspects of diet and eating.

✔ **Occupational therapists:** These staff are involved in preparing patients for a safe discharge home, if possible, by assessing levels of ability and disability and providing adaptations at home if needed; for example, stair rails and raised toilet seats.

(continued)

(continued)

- ✔ **Phlebotomists:** These people take blood from patients so it can be tested in the laboratory.

- ✔ **Physiotherapists:** These provide hands-on treatment and exercises to help with breathing, balance and mobility.

- ✔ **Speech and language therapists:** These therapists offer advice and treatment for problems with speech and swallowing.

- ✔ **Radiographers:** Working in the x-ray department, these staff carry out most of the scans that are then reported on by radiologists (who are doctors).

But knowing a name is different to knowing a person. Get to know the named nurse on admission and use this person as the first port of call to discuss developments in care or problems or concerns you have. Introductions should be easy, because you'll know the nurse's name and face from the time spent with you at admission.

Meeting the junior doctors on the ward may also be possible, because they'll also be around from day to day. Consultants (senior doctors) are a lesser-spotted species who may visit patients on their ward rounds at times when visitors are not permitted and then be in clinics or the operating theatre for the rest of the day. You can always ask to make an appointment with a consultant, however, and he'll be happy to see you either in his office or at the bedside.

See the nearby sidebar 'Who's who in hospital' for a list of all the staff you may encounter.

Taking in Familiar Objects

A few home comforts and familiar objects always make strange, and especially clinical, places seem both less austere and less frightening. Back in 1973, my 6-year-old self was reassured by wearing his own pyjamas, reading a book from home and snuggling up with his teddy at night.

Adults, too, find their own homely items comforting in hospital, although they may not admit it. But most importantly, people with dementia who are prone to heightened confusion in strange and scary environments will certainly be helped by being surrounded by familiar items. Such objects can include anything from pictures to a favourite cardigan.

Offering sources of reassurance

Adopting a British stiff upper lip is all very well when it comes to facing adversity, and your loved one may indeed insist that you don't make a fuss. However, sneaking a few knick-knacks into his hospital case or taking some in the next day will certainly boost his morale.

Here are a few suggestions:

- Framed family photographs
- Pictures of pets
- Favourite blankets from the person's bed or sofa to put over the hospital blanket
- Books he likes to read, including religious texts or cards with verses on if they give him particular comfort
- Puzzle or crossword books if these normally help him fill time, or ask whether you can order a copy of his usual newspaper if he reads one
- A notebook to write reminders on
- His slippers, to make him feel at home
- Make-up bag for women who are never seen without a 'face on'

Remembering that you are what you wear

What people wear can hugely influence their sense of self and their feelings about others. Consider how military uniforms or judges' wigs make you feel. Look at totalitarian regimes that demoralise dissidents by replacing their normal clothes with drab overalls or even stripping them naked.

In the hospital, where everyone is either in a uniform or wearing smart day clothes, patients can also feel inferior if they have to spend all day in a dressing gown, nightie or pyjamas. It certainly reinforces the feeling of a 'them' in charge and a passive, submissive 'us'.

Unless they're due to undergo a surgical procedure or are too ill to care, people don't need to sit about all day in their nightclothes or, worse still, backless hospital gowns. Taking in some normal clothes for a person with dementia to wear in hospital goes some way to normalising the experience for him. Provide a variety of each item – labelled – and enough layers to make sure he's warm. Obviously, you'll have to launder the clothes at home, but it's surely a small price to pay for the reassurance and confidence this simple step should provide.

Visiting Regularly

Your family member, spouse or friend is just in hospital, not prison, and hasn't been kidnapped by time-travelling aliens either. He'll probably enjoy being visited by you. Although visiting hours were traditionally quite restrictive in order to allow the ward to run smoothly and the patients to undergo tests and receive treatment without a crowd of people hanging around, nowadays they're much more flexible, and people with dementia are often given more leeway.

That said, you may of course be an exhausted spouse for whom this time apart, during which you know your other half is being cared for, allows a recharging of the batteries. Or possibly you're a family member or friend, busy with work, children and any number of other things. Perhaps you find the idea of visiting someone in hospital off-putting in itself, because it presents three further potential difficulties:

- ✔ A desire not to get in the way of hospital staff carrying out important tasks
- ✔ A reluctance to enter a building that smells, is full of sick and dying people and reminds you of your own mortality
- ✔ The embarrassing issue of what to talk about after the initial hello and an enquiry about the state of the hospital food

All those things may be true, but for the hospital patient with dementia, regularly seeing familiar faces can be extremely reassuring. And while you're visiting you can provide distraction from the confusion of noise and unknown bustle that's going on around the person morning, noon and night while he sits on the ward.

To avoid the awkward silences so common during hospital visits, consider the following activities to keep you both occupied:

- ✔ Take in family photo albums to go through together.
- ✔ Look through favourite picture books, especially those that help trigger fond reminiscences that you can chat about.
- ✔ Do word or jigsaw puzzles together.
- ✔ If the person is fit enough to do so, go for a wander down the ward, outside to get some fresh air or to the hospital coffee shop.

If you see the hospital admission as a chance for some time out from the tough world of 24-hour caring then try to share visiting duties with friends and family members. Seeing different but also comforting faces still provides reassurance and also much-needed stimulation.

Don't feel guilty if you can't go in to visit every day. If you're already exhausted, trekking back and forth to the hospital won't help. To continue in your role as carer when the person comes home, you need to give yourself time to recover.

Helping at Mealtimes

Another important way in which you can help the person in hospital is to visit him at mealtimes. Although breakfast is often served ridiculously early, you can certainly be there for lunch and dinner. And the nurses will be only too glad of your help.

Helping your relative or friend may only involve collecting his meal and taking it to the table. Cutting it up and even spoon-feeding may also be necessary, however. If you carry out any of these activities, it saves the ward staff a job and allows them to concentrate on other needy patients. Helping with the food also enables you to provide further familiar reassurance to whoever you are visiting and save him the embarrassment he may otherwise feel if someone else has to cope with his coughing, choking or dribbling while eating.

We all deserve to be treated with dignity and respect, and while this is just as likely to be provided by professional nursing staff, there's no substitute for care provided by one of your own.

Chapter 20

Planning for the End of Someone's Life

- -

In This Chapter

▶ Understanding the causes of death in dementia

▶ Describing the people involved in end-of-life care

▶ Deciding whether the person can die at home or needs hospital or hospice care

▶ Allowing the person to die with dignity

▶ Knowing when to let go

- -

Dementia is a progressive illness. And although people may live for many years after diagnosis, the disease is nevertheless known to shorten life expectancy.

There's no way of predicting exactly how long 'someone has left', because it varies depending on the type of dementia, the areas of the brain affected and any other concomitant diseases or illnesses. However, thinking ahead and planning for possible end-of-life scenarios early in the diagnosis is always advisable. You want to ensure that things go as smoothly as possible when the time comes.

Relatives have said to me that they don't want to think about such eventualities at the outset, either because their loved one's death is too painful to contemplate or because they fear that discussing death means they're jinxing the person into dying earlier. I do completely understand that death is always a very difficult subject to consider, but it's something we all have to face.

Everyone strives to live a good and fulfilling life, and by planning end-of-life care it can be possible to help people have a 'good' death too, in peace and with dignity and surrounded by those they love and who love them.

Recognising What Causes Death in People with Dementia

In general terms, of course, people with dementia die for the same reason we all do: none of us are immortal. We're a bit like white goods with built-in obsolescence: the cells and organs in our bodies, like the components of the fridge-freezer, eventually wear out and stop working. That said, some specific aspects of dementia can cause people with this diagnosis to die even earlier.

Effects of dementia itself

People with late-stage dementia deteriorate in a number of ways, both physically and psychologically. Symptoms include

- ✔ Worsening memory
- ✔ Deteriorating speech and ability to communicate
- ✔ Functional declining personal care and hygiene
- ✔ Limited mobility and poor balance
- ✔ Incontinence
- ✔ Difficulties with eating and swallowing
- ✔ Weight loss (caused by the disease itself and not simply reduced calorific intake)

All these changes gang up on people, and their overall health suffers. Malnourishment, aspiration of food into the lungs because of swallowing difficulties and increased risk of falls are common problems, which in turn mean that they can't fight infection easily and are vulnerable to life-threatening, traumatic injuries. (Chapter 5 covers the stages of dementia in detail.)

Effects of other illnesses

As a result of physical deterioration and reduced ability to communicate symptoms to others, sadly people with dementia often succumb to either opportunistic infections or the after-effects of accidents. Paradoxically, they can also be affected by the side effects of medications prescribed to alleviate such symptoms.

Other illnesses and conditions most likely to cause problems are

- ✔ Pneumonia (the cause of death given for two-thirds of people with dementia)
- ✔ Fractures and head injuries resulting from falls
- ✔ Blood clots (deep vein thrombosis and pulmonary embolism) resulting from immobility
- ✔ Severe skin infections caused by pressure sores
- ✔ Kidney disease triggered by poor fluid intake and dehydration
- ✔ Urinary tract infections

Countless other possibilities also exist, all of which can be monitored for and either potentially averted or symptomatically treated with good end-of-life care.

Looking at Who's Involved in End-of-Life Care

End-of-life care can be provided by NHS staff, people employed by local authorities or charitable organisations.

Medical staff

Members of the primary care team generally deliver and co-ordinate end-of-life care. As such, the first port of call for help is the person's GP surgery. It should be possible to arrange for a doctor or nurse to visit the person either at home or in a care home to look at symptoms and treat them as appropriate.

Primary care staff include

- ✔ **GPs:** Try to ensure continuity by involving the doctor who knows the person best. This doctor will be more easily able to monitor changes in the person's behaviour and physical condition and spot and treat any distress. This doctor will also be aware of any advance directives and thus won't initiate intravenous antibiotics or tube feeding, for example, against the person's wishes.

✔ **District nurses and community matrons:** These nurses are well trained in all aspects of end-of-life care. They monitor for changes in condition, liaise with doctors about treatment modifications and arrange for useful aids to be delivered to people's homes to make them more comfortable and to make life for carers more straightforward. Such aids can include hospital beds with special ulcer-preventing mattresses. If someone is already in a nursing home, nurses on site liaise directly with GPs.

Specialist palliative-care teams

Specialist teams of doctors and nurses with expertise in palliative care exist all over the UK. Some are based in hospitals and work with in-patients; others work in the community, often based in hospices. GPs and district nurses make the referral to the palliative-care team and advise on management options. They also visit people in their own homes and deal with families directly.

Involving a palliative-care team shouldn't be seen as 'giving up' on someone; palliative care is there to help make what time that person has left as comfortable as possible and not to hasten death.

Charities

A number of UK charities can offer help, advice and direct support to people with dementia and their carers throughout each stage of the disease. These include

✔ Alzheimer's Society

✔ Age UK

✔ Dementia UK

Contact details for these charities are provided in Appendix A at the back of the book.

Choosing between Home, Hospital and Hospice

Choosing where to die is an important part of end-of-life planning, and people with dementia may want to stipulate their wishes in an advance directive. Alternatively, family members and those with power of attorney may have to decide.

Clearly, circumstances may well dictate that one venue is more suitable than another, but to be honest personal preference and, unfortunately, bed availability win in the end.

Home

Home, sweet home; home is where the heart is; there's no place like home – plenty of phrases highlight the positive attributes of being in your own place. And for many people, home is where they want to end their days – in familiar surroundings and in their own bed. For people with dementia, home offers many other advantages too:

- ✔ They're in a place they recognise.
- ✔ They're surrounded by people they know (even if they don't always recognise them) who can come and go when it's convenient rather than being limited to official visiting hours.
- ✔ Family and friends can be as involved in care as they want or are able to.
- ✔ It's free.

Whatever the person's needs, she can be accommodated in her own home with the help of GPs, nurses, social workers and palliative-care teams. Support can range from providing hospital beds and commodes to professional carers helping with washing and toileting.

Bear in mind that if people have been in a care home for some time, it will be like home to them. They'll be familiar with the surroundings, when cognitive function allows, the staff will know them, and family and friends are likely to be encouraged to be actively involved with care. A nursing home has the added benefit of 24-hour nursing support too.

People who have a significant illness alongside their dementia and have been in hospital as a result can also be discharged from the hospital into a nursing home if they're felt to be at the end of their lives and needing more intensive nursing care than family or intermittent professional carers can provide. This situation will be resolved before leaving the hospital, and the family will be given a choice of available homes.

Hospital

Hospital isn't really the best place for someone entering her last days unless she needs some specialist interventions or treatments that may help control her symptoms. This may be the case for people with dementia who have other conditions such as heart disease, strokes or diabetes.

The benefit of hospitals is, of course, that they provide around-the-clock medical care and excellent facilities for treating illness.

The downsides of hospitals are

- ✔ They're bustling, noisy places with little space for calm.
- ✔ Hospital staff may feel pressured to carry out tests and procedures from which the patient with dementia may not benefit and which may cause the person unnecessary stress.
- ✔ Hospitals have official visiting hours, and families can't just come and go as they please.
- ✔ They're full of ill people with potentially harmful germs that can detrimentally affect those who are run-down and vulnerable, such as those with late-stage dementia.

Avoid hospitals if at all possible. Resist the temptation to dial 999 when a person with dementia develops new symptoms, and phone the GP or community nurse instead. They're just as capable of helping and are unlikely to put someone through the unnecessary upheaval of a trip in an ambulance.

Hospice

Hospices are designed specifically to help manage the symptoms of someone with a terminal illness in a relaxed and calming environment. They aim to offer *holistic* care – that is, treating the person as a whole, physically, psychologically and spiritually. They also provide support for families.

While they do maintain official opening hours, hospices are flexible, especially at the very end of life. They're staffed by specially trained doctors and nurses and so can provide more specialist symptom relief than may be available in extreme circumstances at home. People can be referred to a hospice by GPs, district nurses and nurses from their own palliative-care teams. They're all funded by charity, however, so beds aren't always available immediately.

Ensuring Death with Dignity

Regardless of where it's carried out, the ultimate aim of end-of-life care is ensuring that the person experiences a dignified death. Doctors, nurses and professional carers always do their best to ensure a 'good' death.

Whoever looks after the person with dementia during end-of-life care should be aware of the existence of an advance directive, also known as a living will (Chapter 15 covers these in detail). Once advance directives are made, and as long as they're legal, doctors and nurses have to respect them and the wishes of relatives cannot take precedence. The person with power of attorney should make sure that all medical teams involved in a person's care are aware of the existence and contents of the advance directive and have copies in the medical records.

During end-of-life care, clinical staff focus on making sure that the person seems peaceful and is in as little obvious distress as possible. The person will be washed, moved and medically treated as gently as possible, and every effort will be made to prevent bed sores, discomfort and embarrassment during toileting.

End-of-life care aims to be holistic, focusing on the psychological and spiritual needs of the person rather than concentrating simply on physical factors, as doctors often do. It also allows family members to be involved if they want to be. Death is a normal part of life and should be as non-medicalised as possible.

Understanding What's Involved in Palliative Care

Much of what I cover throughout this chapter makes up the bread and butter of what constitutes palliative care. In this section, however, I sum it up to give you a complete picture of what's involved.

The National Institute for Health and Clinical Excellence (NICE; www.nice.org.uk) defines palliative care as follows:

> *Palliative care is the active holistic care of patients with advanced progressive illness. Management of pain and other symptoms and provision of psychological, social and spiritual support is paramount. The goal of palliative care is achievement of the best quality of life for patients and their families.*

No matter where they're based – hospital, hospice or in the community – all professionals assisting with palliative care therefore have the same aims:

- To help manage distressing symptoms and advise on pain relief
- To treat the patient holistically, dealing with psychological and spiritual issues as well as physical wellbeing
- To offer care and support to families both during the end stages of their loved one's illness and during the early stages of bereavement

Considering what treatments are available

Professionals working in end-of-life care have a large armoury of drugs to use as weapons against the symptoms someone may experience in the last days of life. These medications come in a wide variety of forms so that they can be administered when needed, even if the person has difficulty swallowing or can't take anything orally. Medicines are thus available as

- ✔ Pills
- ✔ Drinkable liquids and suspensions
- ✔ Patches whereby the drug is absorbed through the skin
- ✔ Suppositories (administered rectally)
- ✔ Injections, which can be given under the skin, into muscle or into veins

Medication can be administered for pain, sedation, reduction of anxiety, drying up secretions, to aid sleep, to keep the bowels open and many more symptoms. In short, any medicine for any possible symptom can be made available and given to the patient via the most appropriate route at all times.

Recognising who's who in the team

Palliative care may well be delivered by a GP, with the assistance of district nurses and community matrons who are advised by specialist palliative-care team members. The palliative-care team may also be directly involved, and it includes senior and junior doctors and specialist community nurses. The doctors are likely to be based at either the local hospital or hospice, while the nurses visit people at home.

Palliative care is by no means a nine-to-five job, and as well as providing equipment like beds and commodes to help in the home, hospices and palliative-care teams usually provide 24-hour phone advice and support. Family doctors also give details of people needing end-of-life care to their local out-of-hours GP service, so that calls are prioritised. District nurses are also available around the clock.

Additionally, night-sitters are available. These carers spend the night in the home of the dying person so that their relatives can get some rest and medical intervention can still be summoned if needed. GPs have contact details for this service and can help sort out a referral.

Facing Decisions about Treatment and When to Let Go

Making the decision to let go is never easy. And here I speak from personal experience, having had to sit with a doctor and my mother to discuss the sorts of treatment my father should and shouldn't receive as he lay dying of cancer.

But actually, as his last days went on, those decisions became easier. He was not going to recover, so wouldn't need antibiotics if he had a chest infection; with or without them, we wouldn't get him back. He'd been on medication for blood pressure, an enlarged prostate, high cholesterol and various other long-term conditions, and now no longer needed them.

What we did want him to have was painkillers and medication to relieve agitation, and as he deteriorated these were delivered from a drip through a needle under his skin. We didn't want to lose him, but we knew he didn't have long and wanted him to die in peace.

An advance directive may, of course, contain details of what someone does and doesn't want to be prescribed, which obviously makes things easier, but if not, a pragmatic approach is probably best. Only essential symptom-controlling medicines should be given; everything else can bestopped. And even those that are needed should be given in the least invasive and least disruptive way possible.

Religion, spirituality and end-of-life care

In today's secular society, people may have no faith and no religion and this aspect of palliative care is thus not relevant to them. That may also be true of the clinical teams providing end-of-life care for your loved one. However, if religious practices are an important part of your loved one's life, it's important to communicate that information to the doctors and nurses, who may be so focused on the medical side of things that this aspect of palliative care has slipped from their radar.

Hospitals and hospices have chaplains covering the main faiths, and local vicars, rabbis, priests, imams and so on are permitted to visit. They may also have chapels where services are held and patients can be taken for prayer.

If you want the person with dementia to receive last rites, or you want the funeral to be held quickly for religious reasons, make sure that the people you need to provide these services are alerted in advance. And don't feel embarrassed about making these requests; the nurses and doctors won't feel that you're getting in the way and will be only too happy to make sure they provide the privacy you need.

When it comes to the time of death itself, make sure a 'do not attempt resuscitation' (DNAR) form is in place. Watching someone you love die is intensely painful; no words can describe how it feels. However, allowing the person to slip away quietly in peace is so much better than having paramedics, nurses or doctors jumping on her chest, trying to revive her.

When it's her time, the most loving thing you can do is let her go.

Part V

The Part of Tens

For the top ten tips on how to reduce your risk of developing dementia go to
www.dummies.com/extras/dementia.

In this part . . .

- ✔ Look at some of the best advice for dealing with dementia if you yourself have been given the diagnosis, from discussing the condition with others to managing your work commitments and planning financially for the future.

- ✔ Find out how to be a good caregiver while ensuring that you have time for yourself to recharge your batteries.

- ✔ Discover the truth about some of the most common and misleading myths about dementia.

Chapter 21

Ten Tips for Dealing with Dementia

*H*owever you look at it, being given the diagnosis of dementia is a bit of a hammer blow. And even though you or your close family may have had an inkling that the symptoms you were having might well have been due to this condition, the realisation that you were right all along is still very tough to take.

In the early days after diagnosis, however, you can do plenty to prepare for and even delay the arrival of the condition's later stages and all that can come with them. Here are ten tips to think about putting into action as soon as you can.

Try to Be Accepting of Changes

You'll definitely have started to notice that some things have become more difficult than they used to be. You may be quite forgetful at times and have missed a few appointments or regularly not bought half a dozen items on your shopping list. You may find calculations involving money trickier to work out or get lost when you're out and about, even on well-trodden, familiar routes.

Trying to battle these new difficulties while simultaneously pretending they're not happening inevitably leads to frustration. If you accept your new limitations and work out ways around them with the help of family and friends, you'll feel more in control and will cope better.

The adaptations will be particular to you and won't work otherwise. Consider displaying a wall calendar in an obvious place at home, listing all your activities, so that you don't miss important events. Establish a routine whereby you and the people you live with look at the calendar together at the same time every day. If you're still driving, use a sat nav in the car to prevent getting lost; if you're on foot, use a hand-held sat nav for walkers. Write lists instead of trying to hold things in your head, such as food items you've run out of and people you need to phone. These small steps will make a big difference to your ability to cope.

Let People Know What's Happening

You must tell some people about your diagnosis as soon as possible, such as your boss if you're still working, and the officials at the DVLA if you want to carry on driving. Your boss may be able to organise workplace adaptations to make things easier for you to manage; the DVLA may call you for a practical driving test (see Chapter 10 for details). Beyond that, it's up to you which of your friends, family or workmates to let in on your diagnosis. Health matters are obviously private, and you may not want every Tom, Dick or Harry knowing your most intimate business.

However, telling relevant people yourself has clear benefits:

- ✔ You provide the information on your own terms and give people just the details you want them to know. If they hear it second-hand and in a gossipy fashion, which they no doubt will eventually, they won't get the facts straight and may fill in gaps in their knowledge with all sorts of weird and wonderful theories about what's wrong with you.

- ✔ The more people who know what's going on and how your type of dementia can progress, the more people you have to support you as time goes on.

- ✔ People will be able to make allowances for you when things don't go as they should as a direct result of your condition.

Tell the Driving Authorities

When you're diagnosed with dementia, you need to tell either the DVLA in England, Scotland and Wales or the DVA in Northern Ireland. Failure to inform the driving authorities can result in a whopping £1,000 fine, and if you have an accident without having made such a disclosure you could be prosecuted.

You won't necessarily be told to surrender your driving licence, but you may be asked to take a practical driving test to assess whether you're still safe to be on the road. You may or may not be able to hang on to your licence following the test, subject to regular review. This review involves being sent a short questionnaire by the DVLA to enquire about which doctors and specialist nurses are involved in your diagnosis (so that they can be contacted for information) and ask you questions that check whether your condition is stable or whether further assessment needs to take place.

If you do have to forsake your own wheels at this stage, at least it gives you plenty of time to enquire about other ways of staying mobile, from Blue Badges to bus and train passes.

If your loved one with the diagnosis continues to drive, it's helpful to make sure you experience his driving regularly. While driving with him, ask yourself whether you'd be happy for your children or grandchildren to be in the car with him. If the answer is no or one of hesitation then you need to think further. People often say they only use a car to go down the road, but an accident can happen on your doorstep. It's also better if he chooses to stop driving for himself rather than awaiting his licence to be revoked by the DVLA. A driving licence is such a powerful symbol of independence and being told you can no longer have it can be a crushing blow.

Work Together with Your Partner

If you're in a long-term relationship, working together with your spouse or partner to manage your condition is very important. Don't cut your partner off or, worse still, work against him.

Your spouse or partner may well have thought that you had dementia for some time, but the diagnosis will still come as a shock, and he will have to come to terms with the effects of your illness on your relationship. So be honest with him about your thoughts and feelings about your dementia, and allow him to share his with you. Consider seeing a counsellor together if you need help talking about this difficult subject. Continue doing activities together that you've always enjoyed, and as your symptoms change try new ones that are more manageable but allow you to continue to share the experience.

Sometimes your sexual relationship may be affected, not only by the psychological and emotional effects of the diagnosis but also because of the side effects of any medication you're on. Again, talk about this together and perhaps seek counselling.

Keep Active

Dementia isn't a prison sentence, and you aren't confined within the four walls of your house for the rest of your life. Keeping fit and active is a great way to make sure that your body and brain remain healthy for as long as possible.

If you normally play a sport or go to the gym, keep going for as long as you can (and want to). If you aren't sporty, go for walks or bike rides, or perhaps join a rambling club. Not only will doing so keep you in shape but it will help you meet new people too.

Sort Out Your Finances

When you're newly diagnosed and still fully able to make rational decisions for yourself, spending some time with your family and perhaps an independent financial advisor to review your financial situation is important. You'll then have an up-to-date picture of your income, outgoings and expected expenditure, and thus be in a better place to plan for whatever the future may bring. Simple measures like making sure all your bills are paid by direct debit can make a big difference.

Checking on the various benefits you may be entitled to is also advisable, because you can then begin the application process in good time.

Citizens Advice can advise you on benefits. Go to www.citizensadvice.org.uk or pop into your local branch.

Make a Will

You may think that making a will is a bit morbid, but everyone should have one to ensure that any property, savings or family heirlooms are passed on according to their wishes. Dying *intestate* – without a will – can make it difficult for your relatives to sort things out once you're gone. And in some cases the government will take over and make the decisions for you! Thus, while you still have the capacity to do so, considering who you'd like to benefit from your legacy is a good idea. You may want to include your spouse, children, grandchildren, the local dog rescue centre or the fund for the church roof. Maybe you want to leave instructions for your nearest and dearest to place a plaque in your honour on your favourite park bench. It's your will – you make the decisions.

You can draw up a will yourself without legal help simply by downloading a form from the Internet and filling it in. Alternatively, you can buy a ready-made will from a stationery shop. If you're filthy rich, with the assets to prove it, or want your estate shared out in a complicated way, however, you may want a solicitor to advise you.

Check out the Law Society's website (www.lawsociety.org.uk) for more information.

Look After Your Physical Health

A diagnosis of dementia doesn't mean that your physical health automatically suffers. To remain in the best possible condition

- ✔ Eat a healthy, balanced diet that's low in fat, high in fibre and includes at least five portions of fruit and veg per day. Cut out the chips and pies, and eat your greens.

- ✔ Stay well hydrated by drinking lots of water each day and not too much tea and coffee.

- ✔ Stick to the guidelines for safe alcohol intake; that's two to three units per day for a woman and three to four for a man.

- ✔ If you smoke – stop! Your GP, practice nurse or local pharmacist can provide advice about how to go about it with the best chance of success.

- ✔ Get a good night's sleep and don't nap in the daytime.

Attend Health Checks

The NHS offers free health checks for anyone over the age of 40 to review risk factors for heart disease and stroke. Take up the offer. If you already have ongoing chronic health problems, make sure you attend reviews with your GP and practice nurse. Other checks worth having include

- ✔ Six-monthly check-ups at the dentist to ensure your teeth, mouth and gums remain healthy and pain-free.

- ✔ Annual eye tests at the optician, or more frequently if you have an already diagnosed eye problem.

- ✔ Annual check-up with a chiropodist/podiatrist to make sure that your feet stay healthy and you can thus remain mobile.

✔ A medication review with your local pharmacist. A pharmacist can check on side effects and also interactions between any different pills you're taking. Pharmacists can also arrange for your pills to be supplied in a blister pack to help you remember what to take each day.

✔ A smear test and mammogram (only if you're a woman!). Always go when you're invited, and arrange a new date if you can't make the one suggested.

Having an annual flu jab and the one-off shingles and pneumococcal pneumonia vaccinations is also a smart move. Check with your practice nurse about how and when you can get them.

Continue Hobbies and Pastimes

In short – don't give up. Carrying on doing the things you enjoy doing with your friends and family will do you the world of good. So continue to play golf or bridge, paint or make pots, go train spotting or bird watching, potter in the garden, swim in the local lake all year round, cycle up hills, windsurf, enter your dog or your prize marrows in shows – and get as much enjoyment out of life as possible. You can even take up something new to broaden your horizons and meet new people. In fact any meaningful occupation will assist in keeping your brain active and as able as possible.

If you enjoy travelling and like taking holidays, do that too. If you plan things well enough in advance, you'll always be able to find suitable resorts and hotels.

Chapter 22

Ten Tips for Caregivers, Friends and Families

In This Chapter

▶ Keeping things ticking along as usual

▶ Using professional carers as necessary

▶ Making sure you also look after yourself

*B*eing the partner, friend or relative of someone with dementia often throws you into the role of caregiver. And the closer you are to the person, the more likely you are to be involved.

People with dementia aren't always easy to care for, no matter how much you love them. Unfortunately, dementia not only affects people's intellectual functions like memory and planning, but it also invariably changes their mood and behaviour. And what's more, you may not ever have considered yourself to be carer material in the first place. You may feel that your life is too busy, you don't have the patience and you can't bear cleaning up after other people. But you may nevertheless be thrown, kicking and screaming, into that role.

So here are ten tips for the novice caregiver to help make life not only as easy as possible but also fulfilling.

Make Life as Normal as Possible for as Long as Possible

In the early stages of the disease, soon after someone has been given the diagnosis, she may well be able to continue doing all the things in life she's happily coped with up to this point. She may still be able to go to work, drive a car safely, indulge in her hobbies and get out and about with friends. While this is the case, encourage her to continue. You may need to give a bit of extra help here and there because of the early effects of dementia, but by and large things will carry on for some time as they were: no one goes from diagnosis to total disability in the way that a sports car accelerates from 0 to 60.

Going about her usual life will also help keep her spirits up following the diagnosis of dementia, which can be a crushing blow. So while involving her in decisions about what to do, keep encouraging her to carry on pretty much as normal.

Encourage Her to Plan for the Future

Although you don't wanting the person you're caring for to think the future is inevitably bleak, helping her sort out the financial and legal issues that will ultimately affect her while she still has the capacity to do it for herself is nonetheless a good idea.

The most important issues are

- ✔ **Sorting out finances:** The person with dementia should see a financial advisor to go through her incomings, outgoings and savings, so as to estimate how comfortable she'll be if she retires and what the state may expect her to pay if she needs residential or nursing home care in the future.

- ✔ **Making a will:** Most people have an idea about whom they would like to benefit from their estate when they die and also whom they would like to be the executor(s) of the will. Sorting out these details early on takes a weight off her mind and yours.

  Dying intestate can create huge – and potentially expensive – problems for those left behind.

- ✔ **Setting up direct debits:** The memory problems that affect people with dementia can make remembering when to pay important bills nigh-on impossible. And missing payments may result in having their utilities cut off, for example. If everything's paid by direct debit, there's no risk of this happening, which is one less worry for both of you.

- ✔ **Applying for benefits:** A wide variety of benefits are available for people with dementia and also for their carers. Apply for them as early as possible to receive the maximum advantage. Citizens Advice can advise you on what to apply for (www.citizensadvice.org.uk).

- ✔ **Establishing lasting power of attorney:** People with dementia *must* have someone to manage their affairs when they're no longer able to. Two types of lasting power of attorney exist: one for health and welfare, and the other for property and financial affairs. You don't need a lawyer to set up lasting power of attorney; just download the forms from the government website (www.gov.uk).

Ensure She Remains Healthy

People with dementia need to look after themselves in the same way as anyone else – but you'll probably need to prompt the person you're caring for. First, ensure that she has a healthy, balanced diet, including five portions of fruit and veg a day, plenty of water to drink, not too much fat and alcohol only in moderation. And no smoking. You may have to chip away at the drinking and smoking, and you'll have to be pragmatic about what she eats and drinks as she becomes more severely affected by dementia. Just do your best.

Second, encourage continued exercise. Not only is exercise good for people's cardiovascular health, but it also improves low mood, provides opportunities to socialise and makes people naturally tired, so that they sleep well at night. It's a win–win activity.

Third, you may well need to remind the person you're caring for about basic hygiene. She may need prompting to wash her hands after using the toilet and before preparing food, to change soiled clothes regularly and to brush her teeth at bedtime.

Take Her for Health Checks

One of the many brilliant things about the NHS is its focus on preventive medicine. It provides all sorts of check-ups for vulnerable people to help them remain as fit and active as possible. When someone you care for has dementia, you need to milk this system for all it's worth. After all, you don't get much else free these days.

Ask the person's GP to conduct regular reviews of her general health, and try to stick to the same doctor if possible to ensure continuity of care. If the symptoms of dementia appear to change, see the GP as soon as possible. Practice nurses are also a great resource and will be only too happy to check the person's blood pressure, for example, on a regular basis.

Other professionals who should be involved in monitoring the person's health are the dentist, optician, chiropodist and pharmacist. Finally, ensure the person is up to date with the recommended vaccinations and screening checks such as smears and mammograms.

Consider Underlying Reasons for Changes in Behaviour

As dementia progresses, you'll be presented with a variety of new challenges. Each time you notice a change, however, particularly in behaviour, don't assume it simply results from a worsening of the dementia. A variety of reasons may explain the change, from constipation to loss of hearing, urinary tract infections to an inability of the person to tell you she's in pain.

When communication becomes difficult, people with dementia may express fear, irritability or the reaction to pain by becoming withdrawn and refusing to interact, eat or participate in bathing. Alternatively, they may become aggressive when they're normally placid. If the person you care for behaves differently for no obvious reason, see the GP or dementia nurse to check for underlying physical causes.

Accept Professional Help

As a friend or relative, you may think that all caring responsibilities should fall on your shoulders. Many people feel guilty when they have to enlist outside help or place someone in a care home – but that's what professional carers are for. Think of it like this: getting extra help relieves you of some pressure and frees you to do more things with the person you're caring for that you both enjoy. So consider home care, meals on wheels and home adaptations provided by the local authority, rather than always doing the cleaning yourself, preparing food three times a day and getting out your DIY tools and trying to put up hand rails in your spare time.

Continue to Be Involved When She Enters a Care Home

You obviously don't have to be there 24 hours a day, because that would defeat the object of the person being in a care home and being cared for by someone else. But do help the person become acclimatised to her new surroundings by introducing her to the staff, providing background information on her so that those staff get to know her quickly and bringing in some nick-knacks from home to decorate her room.

Visit regularly and try to take part in any social activities organised by the staff. And don't forget to get grandchildren to visit occasionally too. The presence of children cheers up everyone in the home. Photo boards can also be nice, both in terms of familiarity and reminiscence for your loved one and a window into her life and family for the people now in the caring role. It's important that staff understand at least a little of who the person is, where she came from and what she's enjoyed doing in her life.

Think about End-of-Life Care

Experiencing a good death is as desirable as having a good life, and with planning it can certainly be possible. If the person still has the capacity to make decisions, discuss her wishes with her. If not, talk the matter through with other family members and staff at the care home, if that's where she's living.

Issues you need to consider include place of death, such as home or hospital, and whether the person should be resuscitated if she stops breathing while in an ambulance, for example. The GP will be happy to discuss these matters with you and they can be formalised by signing an advance directive (previously called a living will).

Look After Yourself

Being a carer isn't a nine-to-five job, and it makes emotional as well as physical demands on you. Obviously, if you become ill or burnt out you'll be of no use whatsoever to the person you're looking after. You too should have a healthy, balanced diet, get a good night's sleep, take some exercise, drink sensibly and avoid smoking. If you have ongoing medical problems such as diabetes or asthma, you also need to make sure you attend check-ups and take your medication.

To cope with the emotional and psychological effects of caring, staying in touch with friends you can talk to when things are tough is excellent advice. You can also consider joining a carers' support group. The Alzheimer's Society (www.alzheimers.org.uk) can help you locate a local group and will also provide lots of advice for helping you deal with the strains of caring for someone with dementia.

Finally, if you feel as though you're collapsing under the strain and don't know where to turn, talk to your GP. She'll be able to advise about extra support that may be available to help you and she can point you in the direction of professional counselling and psychotherapy if that's what she thinks you need.

Take a Break

Everyone needs a break sometimes, even people who love their jobs or the person they're looking after. To be able to cope with the demands of caring, it's imperative that you have time for yourself. You need to establish evenings out relaxing with friends, weekend breaks and holidays as crucial parts of your caring timetable. If no one in your family can take over from time to time, you can access day- and night-sitters and also organise for the person with dementia to receive respite care in a care home. Don't feel guilty; time out is essential to your physical and mental wellbeing.

Chapter 23

Busting Ten Myths about Dementia

· ·

· ·

*T*wo types of myth exist: traditional or ancient stories dealing with gods, ancestors and heroes that try to explain a certain worldview or set of beliefs through the characters, and widely held or false notions. In Greek mythology, the tale of Icarus is a good example of the first type of myth. His father, the master craftsman Daedalus, makes wings out of feathers and wax with which he and Icarus can fly. He warns his son not to fly too close to the sun or the sea, but to follow the path he takes as they head off together. Icarus does not listen and flies too close to the sun, which melts his wings and causes him to plummet to his death in the sea. This myth teaches us about the dangers of over-ambition. A four-yearly belief that England can win the World Cup is an example of the second type of myth.

Myths about dementia fall into the second category: they're completely false and misleading and have nothing useful to teach us. In fact, false beliefs have actually led people to try the wrong treatments and avoid seeking appropriate help. Such myths need busting!

All Old People Develop Dementia

Even though the number of people developing dementia is increasing each year and currently stands at 1 in 14 adults over the age of 65, dementia isn't a normal part of ageing. For a start, the statistics tell as that two-thirds of people in that age group don't develop dementia anyway, which busts the myth straight away. On top of that, other triggers are needed to develop dementia, which not everyone experiences. Lifestyle and medical factors such as smoking, poor diet, diabetes, high blood pressure and raised choles-terol play a part; so too do genetics and family history. None of these risks affect everybody.

Thus while older people may be a bit forgetful at times and appear confused about what day it is or the names of their grandchildren, having a few 'senior moments' doesn't amount to dementia. Dementia is a clearly defined medical diagnosis that, thankfully, doesn't apply to everyone.

Dementia Is the Same as Alzheimer's Disease

This myth is like saying that beer is the same as alcohol. It may well be a type of alcoholic drink, but it certainly isn't the only one. Consider wine, gin, tequila, rum, cider, champagne, port and so on. In the same way, Alzheimer's disease doesn't account for dementia in its entirety; rather, it's only one of four main causes of the condition. Although Alzheimer's is obviously the most common and well-known cause of dementia, with its own society to boot (www.alzheimers.org.uk), vascular dementia, fronto-temporal dementia and Lewy body disease also need to be considered. Alzheimer's disease may account for the lion's share of cases (62 per cent), but these other conditions are still responsible for over a third of diagnoses.

Everyone with Dementia Becomes Aggressive

Thankfully, they don't. Anger and aggression can be symptoms of dementia, but they're by no means universal. And why should they be?

We're all capable of being annoyed, losing our tempers and getting stroppy. However, some people are naturally hot-headed and can kick off at the drop of a hat, while others have the patience of a saint and only lose control when they're pushed to the limit. People maintain elements of their own personality even in severe dementia, although that's not to say that disease-triggered disinhibition can't make warlords out of pacifists sometimes. Thus those who were grumpy pre-dementia will often carry on, shouting, cussing and moaning their way through the illness, and mild individuals often remain uncomplaining.

Mostly, however, anger and aggression are displayed by people with dementia when they can't otherwise communicate their discomfort or pain. This behaviour can thus often be prevented by changing something in their surroundings or treating the underlying physical problem.

Dementia Means You'll End Up in a Nursing Home

Two-thirds of people with dementia can safely be looked after in their own homes or those of relatives throughout the duration of the illness according to the Alzheimer's Society (www.alzheimers.org.uk). Sure it can be tough, but with the right input from trained and untrained carers and help from social services it's certainly possible.

Obviously, some people will be so disabled by their condition that their physical and psychological needs become too complex to be managed safely at home. They thus need to be nursed around the clock by professionals. Thankfully, people with such great needs are in the minority.

Aluminium Gives You Dementia

The myth describing a link between dementia and aluminium in cooking pots began in the 1960s when some animal-loving scientists took it upon themselves to inject this element into the brains of live rabbits to see what happened. Not surprisingly, the rabbits fared poorly: they developed protein tangles in their brains, similar to those found in people diagnosed with Alzheimer's disease. Researchers then found high levels of aluminium in the brains of patients with Alzheimer's disease, and a conspiracy theory was born.

No research has corroborated this link, and organisations like the Alzheimer's Society are very keen to dismiss the myth.

The Effects of Dementia Can't Be Alleviated

While it's certainly true – at the moment – that all forms of dementia are both progressive and incurable, it doesn't mean that nothing can be done to ameliorate the symptoms.

First, a handful of drugs are available. They won't stop the condition in its tracks, but they do have the potential to slow its progression. And other medicines can also alleviate some of the more troublesome symptoms. Second, physical and behavioural adjustments can help, ranging from fitting hand rails in the bathroom to psychological techniques to reduce irritability and wandering.

Dementia Is a Hereditary Condition

While some forms of dementia do have a genetic component, it still doesn't follow that the condition runs through families like a bout of diarrhoea after a poorly cooked barbeque. Thanks to the wonders of evolution, disease-bearing genes are watered down when our genes mix with those from people in another family. A healthy lifestyle is also thought to ward off the symptoms triggered by certain genes.

And finally, contrary to the belief held by one of my patients, you can't catch dementia from your grandmother, no matter how much time you spent with her as a child.

Women Are More Likely to Develop Dementia than Men

It is certainly the case that more women than men develop dementia; in fact, the difference in the number of cases of women compared to men increases with age, almost doubling every five years. However, women aren't necessarily more susceptible to the causes of dementia than men. Rather, they tend to live longer (a woman's life expectancy in the UK is 82.7 years compared to 78.9 for a man), thus increasing their likelihood of developing the condition.

If Your Memory Starts to Fail, You're Definitely Developing Dementia

Memory loss is one of the most common symptoms of all types of dementia. But it's by no means the only symptom. To be diagnosed with dementia, people need to demonstrate symptoms affecting not only their cognitive functions (like memory) but also their mood and ability to carry out the normal activities of daily life.

Those who simply start to become forgetful may never develop the other problems and so steer well clear of full-on dementia. Many of these people will instead be diagnosed with mild cognitive impairment. And while it's thought that 10 to 20 per cent of people over the age of 65 develop some degree of mild cognitive impairment, fewer than 50 per cent of them will end up with a diagnosis of dementia.

Red Wine Can Reverse the Effects of Dementia

You may think this myth is purely wishful thinking, but some scientific sense explains it. Red wine contains chemicals called antioxidants, which prevent damage to nerve cells. It's been suggested that antioxidants can thus repair the damage to brain cells that produces the symptoms of dementia. Hence the notion that drinking red wine can 'cure' dementia.

Unfortunately, it's not true! Although the antioxidants in fruit and vegetables may indeed protect nerve cells, no evidence suggests that they can reverse pathological changes in the brain. Rather than warding off or curing dementia, drinking lots of red wine will merely give you a hangover and make your liver beg for mercy.

Appendix A

Useful Contacts and Resources

‫‪•••‬‬

*I*n this appendix I list UK-based organisations that can offer help, advice and support to people with dementia and their carers. Some are UK wide and others are specific to each country in the UK.

Alzheimer's Society

The UK's leading care and research charity for people with dementia and their carers. It provides information and direct support as well as signposting to other helpful organisations.

> Devon House
>
> 58 St. Catherine's Way
>
> London
>
> E1W 1LB
>
> Helpline: 0845 3000336
>
> Website: www.alzheimers.org.uk

Age UK

The country's largest charity supporting people over the age of 60. It offers information, advice and support aimed at ensuring the best possible quality of life for all older people.

> York House
>
> 207–21 Pentonville Road
>
> London
>
> N1 9UZ
>
> Helpline: 0800 169 8787
>
> Website: www.ageuk.org.uk

Carers Trust

Offers quality support, services and training for careers. The free helpline is available Monday - Friday for all Carers to obtain information, advice, and support.

> 32-36 Loman Street,
>
> London SE1 0EH
>
> Helpline: 0800 085 0307
>
> Website: www.carers.org

Carers UK

The national charity supporting and advising carers.

> 20 Great Dover Street
>
> London
>
> SE1 4LX
>
> Helpline: 0808 808 7777
>
> Website: www.carersuk.org

Citizens Advice

This organisation has offices throughout the UK whose phone numbers can be accessed via the relevant websites below. It offers free advice and support on issues ranging from benefits to legal matters.

> 3rd Floor North
>
> 200 Aldersgate
>
> London
>
> EC1A 4HD
>
> Websites: England and Wales – www.citizensadvice.org.uk; Northern Ireland – www.citizensadvice.co.uk; Scotland – www.cas.org.uk

Dementia UK

Dementia UK is a national charity which not only has a helpline offering advice and support for carers, family members, people with dementia and those worried about their memory, but it also provides Admiral Nurses. These mental health nurses provide psychological support to family carers as well as practical advice and information on dementia and how to cope.

Second Floor

Resource for London

356 Holloway Road

London N7 6PA

Helpline: 0845 257 9406

Website: www.dementiauk.org

NHS

The NHS websites offer advice about how to access all local GP and hospital services.

NHS England

Helpline: 111

Website: www.nhs.uk

NHS Northern Ireland

Website: www.hcsni.net

NHS Scotland

Helpline: 111

Website: www.nhs24.com

NHS Wales

Helpline: 0845 4647

Website: www.nhsdirect.wales.nhs.uk

Appendix B

ACE III Exam

The Addenbrooke's Cognitive Examination III (ACE III) is one of the most popular and commonly used tests for dementia in memory clinics and by specialist nurses. It allows them to assess people with memory problems to see whether they're likely to have dementia or not. I've included a copy of the full test here to give you an idea of what's involved.

ADDENBROOKE'S COGNITIVE EXAMINATION - ACE-R
Final Revised Version A (2005)

Name   :
Date of birth :
Hospital no. :

Addressograph

Date of testing: .... /........ /........
Tester's name: ....
Age at leaving full-time education: ....
Occupation: ....
Handedness: ....

ORIENTATION

	Day	Date	Month	Year	Season	[Score 0-5]
➢ Ask: What is the						

	Building	Floor	Town	County	Country	[Score 0-5]
➢ Ask: Which						

REGISTRATION

➢ Tell: 'I'm going to give you three words and i'd like you to repeat after me: lemon, key and ball'. After subject repeats, say 'Try to remember them because i'm going to ask you later'. Score only the first trial (repeat 3 times if necessary).

Register number of trials ......

[Score 0-3]

ATTENTION & CONCENTRATION

➢ Ask the subject: ' could you take 7 away from a 100? After the subject responds, ask him or her to take away another 7 to a total of 5 subtractions. If subject make a mistake, carry on and check the subsequent answer (i.e. 93, 84, 77, 70, 63 -score 4)
Stop after five subtractions (93, 86, 79, 72, 65). ....

➢ Ask: 'could you please spell **WORLD** for me? Then ask him/her to spell it backwards:
....

[Score 0-5]
(for the best performed task)

MEMORY - Recall

➢ Ask: 'Which 3 words did I ask you to repeat and remember?'
....

[Score 0-3]

MEMORY - Anterograde Memory

➢ Tell: ' I'm going to give you a name and address and I'd like you to repeat after me. We'll be doing that 3 times, so you have a chance to learn it. I'll be asking you later'

Score only the third trial

[Score 0-7]

	1st Trial	2nd Trial	3rd Trial
Harry Barnes			
73 Orchard Close			
Kingsbridge			
Devon			

MEMORY - Retrograde Memory

➢ Name of current Prime Minister ....
➢ Name of the woman who was Prime Minister ....
➢ Name of the USA president ....
➢ Name of the USA president who was assassinated in the 1960's ....

[Score 0 -4]

ORIENTATION & REGISTRATION — ATTENTION — MEMORY

ADDENBROOKE'S COGNITIVE EXAMINATION - ACE-R   *Final Revised Version (2005)*

VERBAL FLUENCY - Letter 'P' and animals

➢ **Letters**

Say: 'I'm going to give you a letter of the alphabet and I'd like you to generate as many words as you can beginning with that letter, but not names of people or places. Are you ready? You've got a minute and the letter is P'

[Score 0 - 7]

>17	7
14-17	6
11-13	5
8-10	4
6-7	3
4-5	2
2-3	1
<2	0
total	correct

➢ **Animals**

Say: 'Now can you name as many animals as possible, beginning with any letter?'

[Score 0 - 7]

>21	7
17-21	6
14-16	5
11-13	4
9-10	3
7-8	2
5-6	1
<5	0
total	correct

LANGUAGE - Comprehension

➢ Show written instruction:

[Score 0-1]

Close your eyes

➢ 3 stage command:
'Take the paper in your right hand. Fold the paper in half. Put the paper on the floor'

[Score 0-3]

LANGUAGE - Writing

➢ Ask the subject to make up a sentence and write it in the space below:
Score 1 if sentence contains a subject and a verb (see guide for examples)

[Score 0-1]

ADDENBROOKE'S COGNITIVE EXAMINATION - ACE-R   *Final Revised Version (2005)*

L A N G U A G E - Repetition	
➤ Ask the subject to repeat:**' hippopotamus'; 'eccentricity; 'unintelligible'; 'statistician'** Score 2 if all correct; 1 if 3 correct; 0 if 2 or less.	[Score 0-2] ☐

➤ Ask the subject to repeat: **'Above, beyond and below'**	[Score 0-1] ☐
➤ Ask the subject to repeat: **'No ifs, ands or buts'**	[Score 0-1] ☐▨

L A N G U A G E - Naming

➤ Ask the subject to name the following pictures:

[Score 0-2]
pencil +
watch
☐▨

[Score 0-10]

L A N G U A G E - Comprehension

➤ Using the pictures above, ask the subject to:

- Point to the one which is associated with the monarchy   _____
- Point to the one which is a marsupial   _____
- Point to the one which is found in the Antarctic   _____
- Point to the one which has a nautical connection   _____

[Score 0-4] ☐

L
A
N
G
U
A
G
E

ADDENBROOKE'S COGNITIVE EXAMINATION - ACE-R   *Final Revised Version (2005)*

LANGUAGE - Reading

> Ask the subject to read the following words: [Score 1 only if all correct]   [Score 0-1]

sew

pint

soot

dough

height

VISUOSPATIAL ABILITIES

> Overlapping pentagons: Ask the subject to copy this diagram: [Score 0-1]

> Wire cube : Ask the subject to copy this drawing (for scoring, see instructions guide)   [Score 0-2]

> Clock: Ask the subject to draw a clock face with numbers and the hands at ten past five.   [Score 0-5]
> (for scoring see instruction guide: circle = 1, numbers = 2, hands = 2 if all correct)

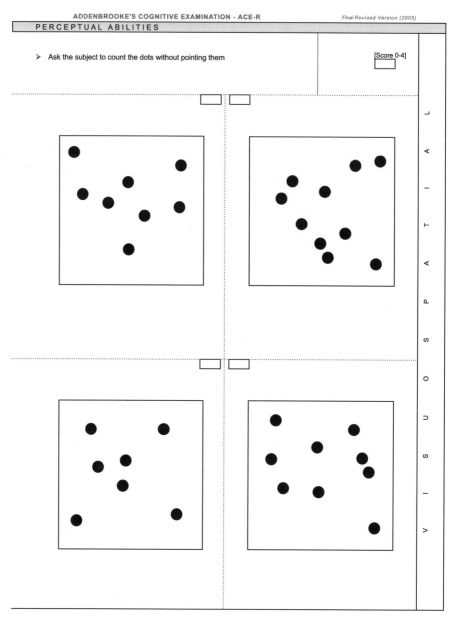

ADDENBROOKE'S COGNITIVE EXAMINATION - ACE-R   *Final Revised Version (2005)*

PERCEPTUAL ABILITIES

➤ Ask the subject to count the dots without pointing them

[Score 0-4]

L A T I A P S O U S I V

ADDENBROOKE'S COGNITIVE EXAMINATION - ACE-R   *Final Revised Version A (2005)*

PERCEPTUAL ABILITIES

➤ Ask the subject to identify the letters   [Score 0-4] ☐

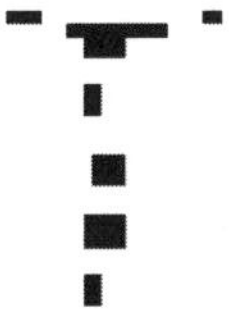

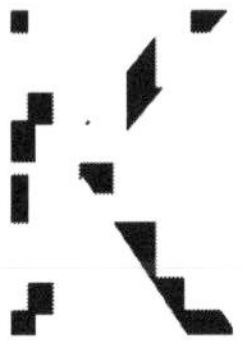

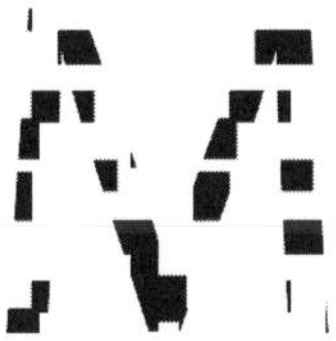

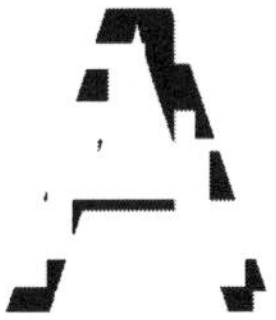

Margin text (vertical): VISUOSPATIAL

RECALL

➤ Ask "Now tell me what you remember of that name and address we were repeating at the beginning'"   [Score 0-7] ☐

	Harry Barnes	....
73	Orchard Close	....
	Kingsbridge	....
	Devon	....

RECOGNITION

➤ This test should be done if subject failed to recall one or more items. If all items were recalled, skip the test and score 5. If only part is recalled start by ticking items recalled in the shadowed column on the right hand side. Then test not recalled items by telling "ok, I'll give you some hints: was the name X, Y or Z?" and so on. Each recognised item scores one point which is added to the point gained by recalling.   [Score 0-5] ☐

Jerry Barnes	Harry Barnes	Harry Bradford	recalled
37	73	76	recalled
Orchard Place	Oak Close	Orchard Close	recalled
Oakhampton	Kingsbridge	Dartington	recalled
Devon	Dorset	Somerset	recalled

General Scores

MMSE	/30
ACE-R	/100

Subscores

Attention and Orientation	/18
Memory	/26
Fluency	/14
Language	/26
Visuospatial	/16

Margin text (vertical): MEMORY   SCORE

Normative values based on 63 controls aged 52-75 and 142 dementia patients aged 46-86

Cut-off <88 gives 94% sensitivity and 89% specificity for dementia
Cut-off <82 gives 84% sensitivity and 100% specificity for dementia

Index

About the Author

Dr Simon Atkins qualified as a doctor in 1995 and has been a full-time GP partner in Bristol since 2000. He holds degrees in Physiology with Psychology from Southampton University and Medicine from Bristol University, and has a master's degree in Science Communication from the University of the West of England.

He has been involved in medical journalism and broadcasting for many years and has been a columnist for the medical magazine *Pulse*, the *Bristol Evening Post* and the *Guardian* as well as contributing to the *BMJ*, the *Observer Magazine* and *FHM Bionic*, *Men's Health* and *Take a Break* magazines. This is his fifth book, having written *Make Me a Baby* for BBC Active and *First Steps to Living with Dementia*, *First Steps out of Smoking* and *First Steps through Insomnia* for Lion Hudson. On television he presented the four-part series *Make Me a Baby* for BBC3 and an episode of *How to Live Longer* on BBC1. He has also appeared regularly on local and national BBC radio discussing health topics.

Simon has a special interest in all aspects of mental health as well as in dementia care, and he is an Honorary Clinical Teacher in Primary Care at the University of Bristol. He is married to Nikki and they have three sons called Harry, Sam and Archie, and a budgie called Frank.

Dedication

This book is dedicated to the memory of my uncle, George Hardyman, and my grandmother, Hilda Taylor, who both experienced dementia first hand.

Author's Acknowledgments

I would like to thank all of the patients with dementia, as well as their families and carers, who I have been involved in looking after during my last 14 years as a GP. It is always extremely tricky working out how best to help people suffering from conditions for which there is no cure, but it is a real privilege to be thought of as someone who can share in their personal struggles and who might even be able to offer help along the way. Thanks also go to specialist memory nurse Beccy Pracownik who has given me much needed advice and support when dealing with these patients and has acted as technical editor for this book.

I would also like to thank my editors, Ben Kemble from Wiley, who commissioned me to write this book and helped me get the process started, and Michelle Hacker my project manager over in Indianapolis who has encouraged me along the way. They have both shown incredible patience when the pressures of my day job have encroached on my writing time and have worked extremely hard to ensure the book has been finished.

And finally thanks must go to my family. Firstly to to my son Sam for drawing the lovely illustrations in the section on how the brain works, but secondly and most especially to my wife Nikki. She is always a great source of support and without her wonderful ability to project manage our three boys and keep the household running smoothly while I beaver away on my laptop, I would have never been able to start, let alone finish, writing this book.

Publisher's Acknowledgments

Project Manager: Michelle Hacker

Project Editor: Simon Bell

Acquisitions Editor: Ben Kimble

Development Editor: Kate O'Leary

Copy Editor: Mary White

Technical Editor: Rebecca Pracownik

Illustrations: Sam Atkins

Project Coordinator: Sheree Montgomery

Cover Image: © iStock.com/peepo

Take Dummies with you everywhere you go!

Whether you're excited about e-books, want more from the web, must have your mobile apps, or swept up in social media, Dummies makes everything easier.

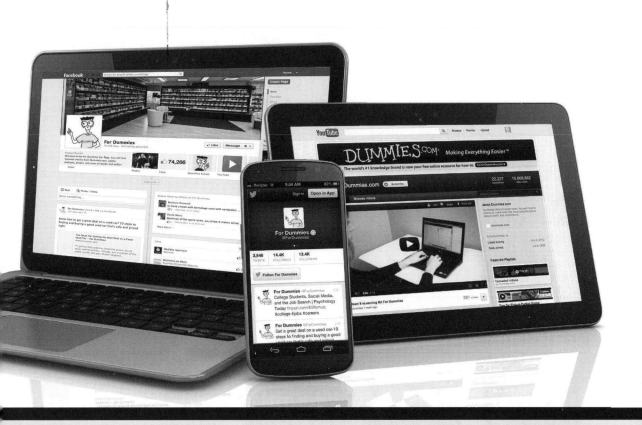

 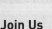
 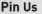

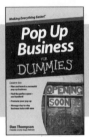

FOR DUMMIES®

A Wiley Brand

BUSINESS

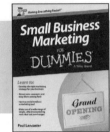

978-1-118-73077-5

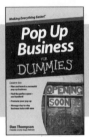

978-1-118-44349-1

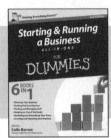

978-1-119-97527-4

MUSIC

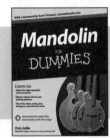

978-1-119-94276-4

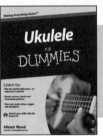

978-0-470-97799-6

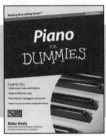

978-0-470-49644-2

DIGITAL PHOTOGRAPHY

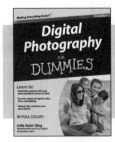

978-1-118-09203-3

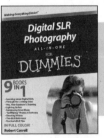

978-0-470-76878-5

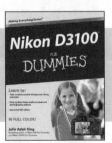

978-1-118-00472-2

Algebra I For Dummies
978-0-470-55964-2

Anatomy & Physiology For Dummies, 2nd Edition
978-0-470-92326-9

Asperger's Syndrome For Dummies
978-0-470-66087-4

Basic Maths For Dummies
978-1-119-97452-9

Body Language For Dummies, 2nd Edition
978-1-119-95351-7

Bookkeeping For Dummies, 3rd Edition
978-1-118-34689-1

British Sign Language For Dummies
978-0-470-69477-0

Cricket for Dummies, 2nd Edition
978-1-118-48032-8

Currency Trading For Dummies, 2nd Edition
978-1-118-01851-4

Cycling For Dummies
978-1-118-36435-2

Diabetes For Dummies, 3rd Edition
978-0-470-97711-8

eBay For Dummies, 3rd Edition
978-1-119-94122-4

Electronics For Dummies All-in-One For Dummies
978-1-118-58973-1

English Grammar For Dummies
978-0-470-05752-0

French For Dummies, 2nd Edition
978-1-118-00464-7

Guitar For Dummies, 3rd Edition
978-1-118-11554-1

IBS For Dummies
978-0-470-51737-6

Keeping Chickens For Dummies
978-1-119-99417-6

Knitting For Dummies, 3rd Edition
978-1-118-66151-2